HMOs
and the Politics of Health System Reform

Joseph L. Falkson, Ph.D.

Published by
American Hospital Association
840 North Lake Shore Drive
Chicago, Illinois 60611
and
Robert J. Brady Co.,
A Prentice-Hall Company
Bowie, Maryland 20715

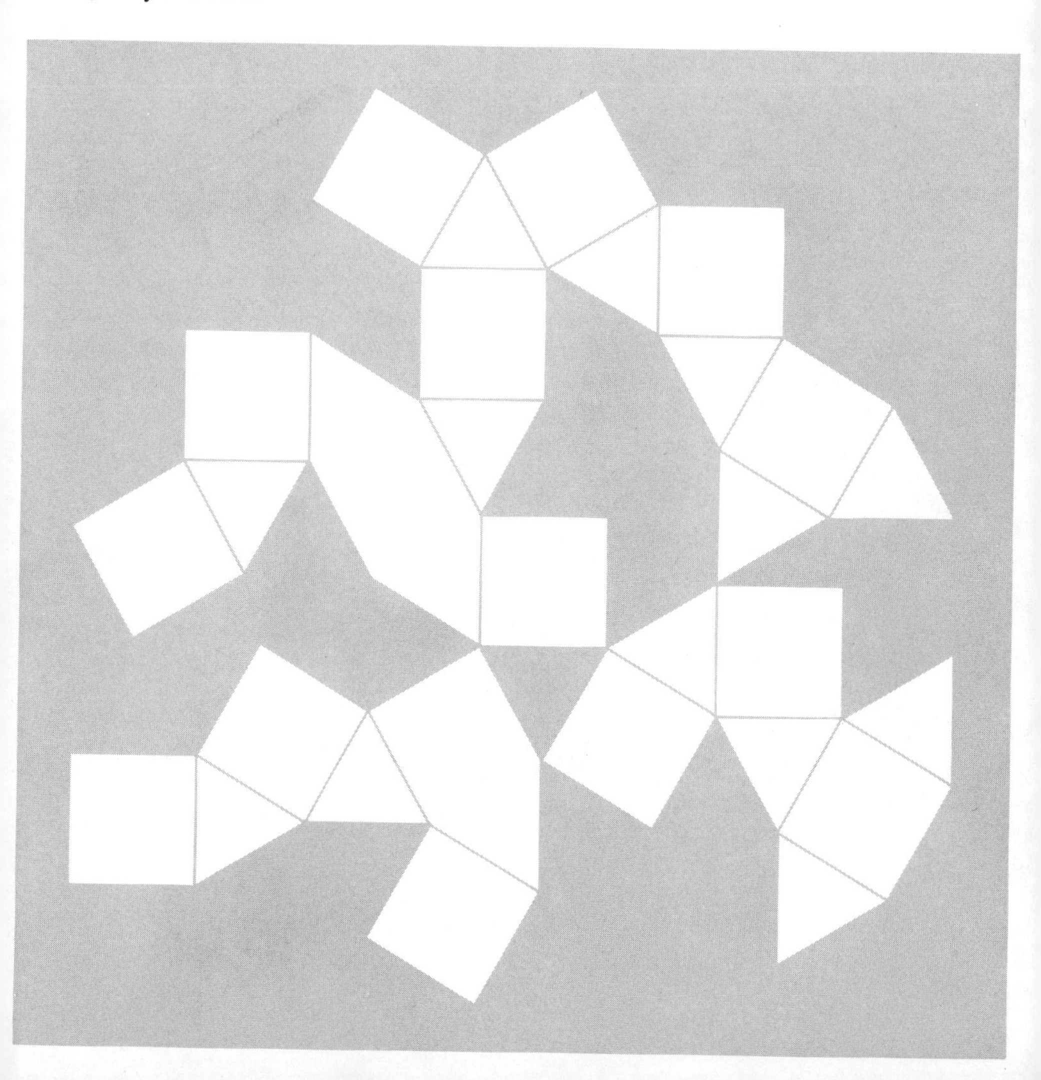

The views expressed in this book are those of the author.

Library of Congress Cataloging in Publication Data

Falkson, Joseph L

HMOs and the politics of health system reform.

Includes bibliographical references and index.
1. Health maintenance organizations — United States.
2. Federal aid to health maintenance organizations — United States. 3. Medical policy — United States.
I. Title.
RA413.5.U5F34 362.1'04'25 79-21932
ISBN 0-87258-288-4
ISBN 0-87258-276-0 pbk.

AHA catalog no. 1183

American Hospital Association
840 North Lake Shore Drive
Chicago, Illinois 60611

Printed in the U.S.A.
1M-12/79-6776

Designed and printed by
Visual Images Inc.
Des Plaines, Illinois

Contents

Foreword

Scholarly analysis of the politics of health policy is no longer a novelty. But when such analysis is focused on as important a new direction — in health care delivery and federal policy — as health maintenance organizations (HMOs), we should be especially grateful for it.

The nation continues to aspire to better health status and to struggle with its health problems. What to do, as a matter of national health policy, to enhance the possibility of meeting agreed upon objectives remains frustratingly difficult. This is true even though some formidable barriers to policymaking at the national level have been removed. For example, not many years ago there was perceived to be broad constitutional inhibitions against the federal government's pursuing an activist role in the promotion of the people's health. Gradually, since the end of World War II, such proscriptions have dropped away. No longer are such limited activities as biomedical research support and grants to states for building hospitals the only acceptable federal functions. Now, the government even pays for health care for large numbers of citizens, particularly the aged and the poor. The principal new barrier to further enlargement of the federal role in health is a fiscal one.

Fiscal concerns, and a new tentativeness on the part of policymakers about whether proposed programs are certain to bring desired results, have combined to keep national health insurance in an elusive status. Indeed, despite much talk and continuous planning, national health insurance remains a perennial ghost among the statutes that together make up national health policy.

In the past decade, the few new health policy initiatives to be taken by the federal government (for example, health planning and professional standards review organizations) have had, as a fundamental aim, controlling unrestrained growth, whether in proliferation of services and facilities or costs. Only one of them, that involving the promotion of HMOs, has within it the potential of significantly altering patterns of health care delivery in the United States. This is one of the reasons Joseph L. Falkson's book is an important one.

In his lively account of the emergence and maturing of the HMO concept as a new approach to health care and to national health policy, Dr. Falkson also helps us to understand both the impulse of decision makers "to do something" that might advance us toward our goal of better health, and the constraints on what they might soundly do, given conflicting priorities, splintered constituencies, and tight budgets. Dr. Falkson shows us, through fresh and fascinating illustrations, how difficult and elusive the search for national health policy has been over the past decade. His detailed and copiously documented analysis of why successive Republican and Democratic administrations came to focus on HMOs as one important cornerstone of their national health policy offers important insights, both into the nature of national leadership in health affairs and the labyrinthine pathways through which successful policies must travel. What is most striking is the high probability for failure of most new ideas that seek to challenge conventional nostrums and entrenched prerogatives. Dr. Falkson's account of the troubled journey of HMOs through the national health policymaking process is testimony enough to the durability, vitality, and permanence of prepaid health care on the nation's agenda of significant social reforms.

Stephen P. Strickland, Ph.D.
Vice-President
Aspen Institute for Humanistic Studies
Washington, DC
December 1979

Preface

This book describes the evolution of the federal government's commitment to prepaid health care in the United States in the 1970s. Three presidents and three Congresses have endorsed the concept of prepaid health care, or health maintenance organizations (HMOs), albeit with differing levels of enthusiasm. It would be the ultimate in understatement to conclude that HMOs have displayed a good deal of resiliency in the face of entrenched and powerful opposition. In fact, the sustained and largely continuous support provided by various presidents and Congresses has been altogether singular precisely because of the determination of opponents of HMOs. Why HMOs came to play so important a role in national health policy and how the federal commitment was sustained and nurtured are the main subjects of this book.

In a very real sense, the genesis of this study parallels the evolution of federal HMO policy. The idea for the study evolved during the summer of 1971 while I was searching for materials to use in a new course on health policy and politics that would be offered to my students at the University of Michigan that fall. In pursuing my search, I had occasion to meet the (then) associate administrator for planning and evaluation of the (now defunct) Health Services and Mental Health Administration, Beverlee Myers.

Myers introduced me to a fascinating story: how health maintenance organizations had become the central feature of the Nixon Administration's national health strategy. A number of additional meetings with her led to my writing a short paper on the "Origins of the Health Maintenance Policy," which I subsequently used as the basis for a series of lectures and to show to people whose advice I solicited on the potential of the HMO story for a book.

By the fall of 1972, I had received sufficient encouragement from major figures in the HMO movement to begin a serious search for support of a book-writing project on HMO politics and policy development. An award from the Robert Wood Johnson Foundation made it possible to begin work over the summer of 1973. Research proceeded slowly but — I believe — thoroughly, with periodic interruptions for other assignments, over the next five years, and materials were continuously updated as new events unfolded. The result is the present analysis, describing HMO politics and policies through mid-1979.

I have interviewed more than 50 people in the course of my research — virtually all of the key actors in the national HMO policymaking process. These individuals were extraordinarily generous in providing me with complete access to their HMO files, which ultimately amassed to nearly two full filing cabinets of fascinating notes, memorandums, and working papers. These documents, coupled with the interviews, have enabled me to piece together the events surrounding the formulation and evolution of HMO policies in great detail.

The book has three objectives. First, I have sought to present a factual account of the emergence of the health maintenance strategy and HMO program as centerpieces of national health policy in the 1970s. Second, I have tried to describe the congressional and health interest groups' attempts to shape a health maintenance policy in their own images. This analysis offers important insights into institutional and ideological cleavages that have tended to constrain the making of national health policies throughout the present decade. And third, I have attempted to offer insights into future directions for HMO policies and to place them within the broader framework of national health policy.

The usual caveats about case studies are in order to the reader of this volume. Although seminal themes about American politics and policymaking are inextricably part of the study of HMO policy, I have consciously chosen not to ponder long on these "great themes" of American politics as they may or may not pertain to the flow of events described. I have left much, therefore, to the speculation of a thoughtful readership, which may choose to array the facts of HMO politics and policymaking within any one of a number of available paradigms and models of the American system of public policymaking. For my part, I have tried to tell an interesting and compelling story, one that will, I hope, fascinate both the casual and sustaining observer of the nation's health affairs. Large generalizations and broad conclusions, therefore, are probably beyond the scope of this work. A comparative analysis of the two or three other major health policies that emerged during the same period would disclose the extent to which the present political history of HMOs was part of a larger pattern of stable institutional processes. That is another study.

Acknowledgments

This project benefited from the support and counsel of many people. Some of them require special mention because they took an interest in me and my work very early on: Beverlee Myers, who supported the project first; Paul Ellwood, who kept impeccable records of the HMO policy's earliest history and who shared them with me; James Doherty, who painstakingly recounted, with his amazing memory, a dazzling array of seemingly obscure events and meetings and placed them in broad and comprehensive perspective; and Frank Seubold, with the federal HMO program almost from the beginning, who provided a lively and detailed account of the uneven passage of HMO through HEW's permanent health agencies and who also reviewed the draft manuscript with diligence and wit. There were many others. I am deeply grateful for their cooperation and patience.

A special note of thanks must be reserved for James E. Bryan, who brought a rare combination of skill and experience to the task of editing this volume. Jim had served for a time as the Washington representative of the American Association of Foundations for Medical Care. Although he had not been active in HMO politics for some years, when I asked him to help me in the spring of 1978, Jim's earlier experiences enabled him to comment critically on the content, as well as on the style, of the manuscript. I am grateful for his discipline in pointing out ways to delete extraneous materials that tended to detract from central ideas and themes.

CHAPTER 1

The Search for National Health Policy

Crises create possibilities for change. Whether the focus is the individual, the family, the community, or the nation, it is fear of pending catastrophe or belated response to one already arrived that motivates people to strong individual or collective actions. The New Deal was President Franklin D. Roosevelt's immediate response to the collapse of the American market economy. The Marshall Plan was President Harry S. Truman's answer to the economic chaos in Western Europe following World War II. The crisis in health affairs, however, lacked the urgency of those earlier challenges. It came upon the nation slowly, and its effects were just beginning to become apparent toward the close of the past decade.

The Health System in Crisis

By 1969, some thoughtful observers of national health affairs were looking at the persistent and steep inflation in the health sector of the economy with mounting trepidation. The general public, however, was blissfully unaware of the mounting crisis. For, unlike the period of Depression beginning in 1930, an intricate network of public-private health insurance masked the true dimensions of the economic crisis from the bulk of the civilian population.

Medicare and Medicaid were the immediate focus of attention. Essentially open-ended federal commitments to underwrite health care for the aged and the eligible poor by guaranteeing payments to hospitals on a cost-incurred basis and to physicians on a "usual, customary, and reasonable" fee-for-service basis, Medicare and Medicaid were powerless either to regulate the flow of payments in the fee-for-service system or to ensure that adequate health services would be available to meet swelling demands from expanded entitlements. Government spending for Medicare and Medicaid was easily identifiable as a significant contributor to the rapid inflation in health care costs between 1966 and 1969. These new entitlements, however, were not the only inflationary forces at work. Other, more ominous sources of inflation could be identified.[1]

The Senate Finance Committee staff, early in 1970, noted that all early actuarial projections of Medicare program costs had grossly underestimated actual experience. When new projections had been made on the basis of the first two years of Medicare program experience, the results again were staggering:

---

1. Because the sharp rise in the rate of growth in hospital costs between 1966 and 1969 coincided with the advent of the Medicare and Medicaid programs, many thoughtful analysts would draw the conclusion that the latter "caused" the former. This causal inference was, in fact, drawn by the Senate Finance Committee in 1970. Their conclusion that the reason for the association was rooted in expanded eligibility and benefits, however, greatly oversimplified the complex relationships involved. See: "Medicare and Medicaid: Problems, Issues, and Alternatives," Report of the Staff to the Committee on Finance, U.S. Senate, Feb. 9, 1970.
   Others — Louise B. Russell of the Brookings Institution, in particular — have provided a more complex and persuasive explanation with the benefit of a decade or more of data at their disposal:

   > From 1950 to 1965 cost per patient day in short-stay hospitals grew at an average rate of 7 to 8 percent a year. . . . Three to 4 percent was attributed not to higher prices and wages, but to the growing amounts of resources — labor, equipment, and supplies — used per patient day. . . . The rate of increase in the resources used per hospital day jumped to an average of 6 percent a year with the advent of Medicare and Medicaid. While the exact share of cost increase attributable to increasing input levels has varied from year to year, the accumulated growth over the decade [since the advent of Medicare and Medicaid] has resulted in a level of inputs used per patient day that is almost 80 percent higher than the level of 1966. [Russell, pp.180-181]

   In other words, Medicare and Medicaid accelerated the rate of increase of capital inputs that went into the production of discrete units of service output. The major effects of Medicare and Medicaid, therefore, were upon the supply of health resources rather than upon the demand for health care services. Instead of accelerated demand, the reason for this effect, or "cost push" inflation, may be traced to the cost reimbursement nature of hospital insurance, which, in effect, treats health resources as "free goods."

> The increase in projected program costs was dramatic. The cost was now estimated at 1.79 percent of taxable payroll over the next 25 years; 1970 benefit payments were estimated at $5,029 million, and 1990 benefit payments were projected at $16,380 million — in both cases, almost twice the original estimates.[2]

Both the newly elected Nixon Administration and the Democratically controlled Congress had arrived at a crossroad with regard to federal health policy in 1969. The economic situation made it imperative for additional responses from the federal government. Those responses, however, would somehow have to shape into a coherent system over 20 years of federal health programs designed to expand the stocks of the nation's health resources and to broaden access to care for many needy groups. For, in reality, the federal government's fragmented and strategically uncoordinated investment policies were themselves inflationary. Now, under a new Administration, a heretofore untried discipline and restraint was the next order of business.

The Republican Perception of the Health Crisis

Both Democrats and Republicans sought to capitalize on the crisis in health care costs — in their own ways and in conformance with their own ideological commitments. Liberal Democrats rallied behind the newly formed Committee for National Health Insurance, led by United Auto Workers chief Walter Reuther and Sen. Edward M. Kennedy (D-MA). In the summer of 1969, they were hard at work on a comprehensive, govenment-financed health insurance program. Their proposal, the Health Security Program, was submitted to Congress in September 1970 as the most liberal response to increasing congressional interest in finding solutions to the health crisis.

The Republicans were to look for their own solution in directions other than national health insurance (NHI). Republicans usually seek

---

> According to this explanation of the growth in costs, Medicare and Medicaid are only part of a larger problem. They accelerated the transformation of medical care, which was already well under way, from a market in which patients and doctors faced prices that were reasonable indicators of the resource costs of their decisions to one in which — particularly where hospital care is covered — prices have been nearly eliminated [Russell, pp. 182].

See: Louise B. Russell. Medical Care Costs. In: Pechman, Joseph A., editor. *Setting National Priorities: The 1978 Budget*. Washington, DC: The Brookings Institution, 1977, pp. 177-206.

2. "Medicare and Medicaid: Problems, Issues, and Alternatives," Report of the Staff to the Committee on Finance, U.S. Senate, Feb. 9, 1970, p. 30.

solutions to economic problems by attempting to reduce inflationary pressures, which, they argue, result from too much government spending. This means that Republicans, for political purposes, must find ways of glamorizing policies that are basically reactive or reconstructive rather than aggressively innovative.

The Nixon Administration had come to office in January 1969 with few commitments to fulfill in domestic policy, and health policy was not of preeminent concern to the White House staff. Although President Richard M. Nixon, as his first executive act, on January 23, 1969, set up an impressive array of issue-oriented subcommittees under his Urban Affairs Council, none of these was specifically charged with health policy. [3] It was not until much later in 1969 that the White House, belatedly realizing that health had been ignored, scheduled a Presidential health initiative.

Aside from health being overlooked when the Urban Affairs agenda was drawn up, the Nixon initiative in this field was balked by the "Knowles affair." When Robert Finch, Mr. Nixon's closest political adviser, was appointed Secretary of Health, Education, and Welfare, he delegated to John G. Veneman and Lewis H. Butler, his two top aides, operational responsibilities for organizing health and welfare activities in HEW. Butler was responsible for health, while Veneman worked on welfare. For Butler the health assignment was to be temporary until a new Assistant Secretary of Health and Scientific Affairs could be recruited, and that became his first task in early 1969. Finch, Veneman, and Butler could not then have known that they were about to be entangled in an intrigue that would throw the early months of the Administration's health policy process into total disarray.

Shortly after taking office, Finch decided to appoint John H. Knowles, M.D., then general director of the Massachusetts General Hospital, as the Assistant Secretary for Health and Scientific Affairs. The decision profoundly affected the course of health policy development in the early Nixon Administration because Finch failed to get Knowles approved. Knowles's appointment hovered in limbo for nearly six months as Finch vainly sought to secure political clearance for his designee.[4] By June,

---

3. The subcommittee assignments were: future of the model cities program, minority business enterprise, welfare, crime, voluntary action, internal migration, surplus food and nutrition, mass transit, and transition to peacetime economy at the end of the Vietnam hostilities.

4. More specifically, the American Medical Association had expected to exert a strong, if not decisive, influence in the naming of the new Assistant Secretary. Knowles, a liberal and iconoclastic member of the medical establishment, was clearly an unacceptable

however, the now infamous Knowles affair had made the appointment hopeless, and on July 10, 1969, Nixon, along with Finch and Veneman, presented their fallback choice, Assistant Secretary-designate Roger O. Egeberg, M.D., to the public. Egeberg was hastily recruited from his deanship of the University of California-Los Angeles (UCLA) Medical School when it was apparent that Knowles would not be recommended.

The long, unsuccessful struggle to appoint John Knowles left a critical gap in the ranks of HEW's health leadership at a time of new and perplexing problems. Federal health leadership, in short, was left to the control of two progressive "civilians," Veneman and Butler, rather than to a physician. The locus of power in HEW health affairs shifted to the office of the Assistant Secretary for Planning and Evaluation and to the Under Secretary's office, where nonphysician professionals, for example, Ph.D.s, management specialists (MBAs), and lawyers, took the lead in making national health policy rather than the traditional health professionals who staffed the U.S. Public Health Service. These new federal health policymakers possessed the analytical skills to address the essentially economic problems plaguing the health system. For, in fact, the problems facing the federal health establishment were more in the realm of politics and economics than medicine. And, over the ensuing decade, as the economic imperative relentlessly dictated, the erosion of medicine's dominance in national health affairs also continued. Policy initiatives, once lost, are difficult to recover.[5]

The disarray in HEW's health policymaking apparatus, highlighted by the Knowles affair, also placed the Administration far behind the liberal Democrats, led by Kennedy, in the generation of national health policy initiatives. The formation of the Committee for National Health

---

choice to the AMA, which expressed its displeasure through the Senate minority leader, Everett M. Dirksen, and Rep. Bob Wilson, the head of the Republican Congressional Campaign Committee. These powerful Republican leaders articulated their opposition to Knowles directly to the White House, thereby effectively blocking Finch's effort to get Dr. Knowles appointed.

5. There was some indication, eight years later, that the initiative had yet to be recovered. In 1977, the entering Carter Administration could only get its third choice for the job of Assistant Secretary for Health (ASH) to accept the assignment. He lasted only about six weeks in the tentative capacity as "assistant secretary-designate" and was never permanently appointed. A permanent ASH was not found until June, when Julius Richmond, M.D., agreed, reluctantly, to take the job. Moreover, the reorganization of March 1977, which set up a Health Care Financing Administration, further reinforced the weakness of the ASH by creating yet another powerful health agency that reports directly to the Secretary, not to the ASH.

Insurance in late 1968, with Kennedy as a member, only dramatized the Administration's vulnerability on the health front.[6] The Administration was sharply criticized by the media for not offering significant health policies during its first six months in office. By the spring of 1971, therefore, it belatedly moved health to the forefront of critical policy concerns.

The stage was set for a major initiative in health policy. The situation facing the Administration in the health policy arena in early July 1969, however, was decidedly bleak. The Administration was unable to complete its health policy appointment roster. It was outflanked on the left by the labor-liberal coalition, the Committee for National Health Insurance. It was being sniped at from the Hill and faced a debilitating national inflation in health care costs, the primary cause of which was, in its eyes, the Medicare and Medicaid programs inherited from the Johnson Administration. Action, or the appearance of action, was the order of the day.

* * *

On July 10, 1969, Nixon held a press conference in the Roosevelt Room of the White House. The President presented his designated Assistant Secretary for Health and Scientific Affairs, Roger Egeberg, under conditions intentionally stage-managed to foster the impression of an Administration diligently pursuing the formulation of a national health policy. The President opened the news conference by declaring:

> When this Administration came into office in January, we initiated a major study of the nation's health care problems and programs. . . . The report that I have received from Secretary Finch and Dr. Egeberg indicates that the problem is much greater than I had realized. We face a massive crisis in this area and unless action is taken both administratively and legislatively to meet that crisis within the next two or three years, we will have a breakdown in our medical care system which could have consequences affecting millions of people throughout this country.

---

6. See chapter 5, pp. 115-120, for an account of Kennedy's aggressive efforts, throughout 1970 and 1971, to push liberal solutions forward. The senator's difficulties in making progress on the national health insurance front led directly to his evolving interest in HMOs, by mid-1971, much to the alarm of Administration HMO advocates.

The report Nixon alluded to used equally hyperbolic language. The President picked up the term *breakdown* from the report, although the term *crisis* appears to have been his own. The report focused on

> . . . a crippling inflation in medical costs causing vast increases in government health expenditures for little return, raising private health insurance premiums and reducing the purchasing power of the health dollar of our citizens.[7]

Nixon's declaration was a singular event. It showed not only that all major political factions had discovered that something was indeed very wrong with the health system, but also, more remarkably, that a Republican administration widely believed to be passive on social issues was actively seeking solutions.

The Nixon Administration sought, throughout that eventful July day, to distinguish its own analysis of the nature of the health crisis from that of congressional Democrats. The problem was articulated in terms of mounting inflation forcing great numbers of Americans out of the health care market each year. The solution was to bring that inflation under control by limiting price increases, thereby increasing consumer purchasing power. National health insurance, the Democrats' solution, was seen as an improper, short-run palliative that would only fuel the superhot health economy at a time when it needed to be cooled down. So, the President would not propose NHI at that time, but would seek to improve the cost-effectiveness of extant programs, such as Medicaid, to improve the health system's productivity and efficiency.

This response was both good politics and good Republican economics. The Administration would urge health system reform while the "spendthrift" Congress would continue to advocate outmoded "throw money at the problem" approaches, particularly in its call for NHI. The President's advisers appeared to realize that unless basic changes were made in the structure of the health system itself, federal dollars would only aggravate rather than correct the underlying problems. The system of financing health care was the major culprit. So, federal solutions that merely offered to put more money into that system would in the final analysis fail.

The Medicaid program was singled out for particularly harsh criticism:

---

7. Robert H. Finch, Secretary of HEW, and Roger O. Egeberg, M.D., Assistant Secretary-Designate for Health and Scientific Affairs, *A Report on the Health of the Nation's Health Care Systems*, HEW/Office of the Secretary, July 10, 1969.

> Badly conceived and badly organized, the Medicaid program has attempted to provide medical services for the poor by pushing them into the Nation's already overburdened health care system without developing the capacity in the system to serve them and without building the capability in the states to manage the program.

The report and press conference, then, were designed to recover some of the initiative lost during the long, crippling Knowles affair. The emphasis on the failures of existing governmental programs recast the "health problem" in terms appealing to a Republican Administration: the problem was not that government was not doing enough; rather, government was doing quite enough, and rather poorly at that. In this way, the report attempted to respond to pressure from the Senate Finance Committee, highly critical of the management of the Medicaid program. Only nine days before, on July 1, Veneman had concurred with the Finance Committee that the executive branch had been doing a poor job in Medicaid management:

> Sen. Jordan: Now, with respect to Medicaid, our staff review made this statement, and I would ask you to comment on it:
>
> "Federal officials have been lax in not seeing to it that states establish and employ effective controls on utilization and costs. . . . The federal Medicaid administrators have not provided states with the expert assistance necessary to establish and implement proper control. . . ."
>
> . . . What is your answer to this charge?
>
> Mr. Veneman: I would agree with the charge, Senator.[8]

Similarly, the report obliquely answered critics who believed more money should be spent through NHI. While recommending a number of administrative and legislative proposals to tighten control over Medicare and Medicaid, it carefully avoided mention of NHI. Instead, the focus was on cost containment measures to be applied to the two programs and on "greater flexibility to engage in incentive reimbursement and demonstration projects." The report also declared: "We will move in the direction of reducing the Medicaid burden on general revenues by shifting to various forms of prepayment." For the moment, the Administration intended only to experiment with incentive reimbursement, not to implement such a program on a nationwide basis.

---

8. John G. Veneman, testimony before the Committee on Finance, U.S. Senate, July 1, 1969.

The discussion in the press conference then turned to prepayment. Veneman spoke of prepayment in the context of the medical care foundation plans, such as the San Joaquin Medical Foundation; he mentioned group practices in the context of incentive reimbursements that would allow them to retain a portion of what they were able to save below the average cost of Medicaid. Most significantly, incentive reimbursement and prepayment were not linked conceptually. Both were seen as fiscal experiments, along with a laundry list of other "interesting" cost control ideas. All of the basic conceptual elements of health maintenance were present in that July meeting: prepayment, foundation medical plans, group practice, and incentive reimbursement. However, the framing of all of these concepts into a comprehensive health system plan called the health maintenance strategy would not occur until the following February.

The immediate task in July 1969 was to gain control over exploding Medicare-Medicaid costs. Hence, the Administration's initial health policy focus was on cost containment as a way to improve health system productivity. The Democrats' alternative, expanded investment through an NHI program, was dismissed as inflationary. It all made good sense, both politically and economically.

A Presidential Health Message Is Scheduled

A health work group was established in the White House during the fall of 1969 to begin planning for a major Presidential health message, which could be delivered in early 1970. The work group consisted of the same people organized to plan a higher education message: Lewis Butler, chairman; Edward Morgan, deputy counsel to the President; Herbert Stein, of the Council of Economic Advisors; Richard Nathan, assistant director of the Office of Management and Budget; Martin Anderson, deputy to Presidential counsellor Arthur Burns; and Chester Finn, deputy to Presidential assistant Daniel P. Moynihan. Throughout the fall, however, no work was accomplished on the health message, as work proceeded on higher education.

In a memorandum to Presidential adviser John Ehrlichman in early December, Butler summarized the Administration's frustration in trying to articulate a health policy to serve as the basis for a Presidential message:

> A number of well-publicized groups are advocating universal health insurance (Reuther's Committee of 100, Governor's Conference, etc.). Whatever form such a plan might take, the cost would be in the

> range of $20 billion annually. More important, increasing the demand on our overstrained medical facilities and manpower would, at this point, almost literally collapse the system.[9]

Then, reaching for the only positive proposal yet articulated by the Administration, Butler reiterated "that ultimately some kind of national health insurance system should be enacted, but the immediate problem is to train more doctors and subprofessional people, and get away from hospital-dominated care into more efficient systems." How these things were to come about was not spelled out. All that could be concluded, in fact, was that:

- The enormous inflation in medical costs means that we are buying little if anything more for the enormous annual increases in the cost of Medicaid and Medicare.
- The NHI system would fuel this inflation beyond all control.
- The critical need now is to change the system to get more and different kinds of manpower to increase our capacity to deliver medical services.

Coming up with policy positions to address these problems was an exceedingly elusive undertaking. Butler and his staff struggled to articulate a coherent series of policies throughout January 1970. In early February, Butler presented to the White House health work group a memorandum he hoped would "help us start our discussions on the financing portion of a possible health message."[10] Under the heading "Alternative Plans for Financing Health Care" appeared the following options:

- Maintain the status quo
- Expand the current public programs
- Change the nature of Medicaid
- Extend and improve private health insurance
- Provide new public mandated and/or subsidized programs

Other suggestions for structuring a health message were presented to Butler by Arthur Hess, deputy commissioner of the Social Security Administration. Hess offered a succinct restatement of problems facing health and medical care and a review of possible options, which, unlike earlier presentations to Butler, began to outline some concrete delivery system choices. Hess specifically linked federal financing arrangements to

---

9. Lewis H. Butler, memorandum for John D. Ehrlichman, draft, HEW, Dec. 10, 1969.
10. Lewis H. Butler, memorandum for members of the Health Group, Office of the Assistant Secretary for Planning and Evaluation, HEW, Feb. 10, 1970.

potential delivery system outcomes, and he suggested some parameters within which to structure concepts:

- Strengthening financing to bring about a balance between capacity and demand
- Regulating public and private financing and use of reimbursement formulas to improve the supply, use, efficiency, and productivity of health care service.[11]

Butler's frustration with his failure thus far to come up with a health policy (and his prescience as to the course of events in the '70s) is reflected in his response to Hess:

> I find little, if anything, to disagree with in your memo of February 4. It seems our course should be:
>
> 1. To educate those in the White House about the intricacy of the health industry and the fact that no simple solutions are at hand,
> 2. To prepare them, and the public, for, say, a 10-year period in which adjustments will be made in the "system," many of which will not have an impact for a long time; and
> 3. To offer proposals now which, while they do not promise quick solutions, can be seen as major steps toward the kind of ultimate organization and delivery that we all want.
>
> From talking with various reporters and others, I am impressed that they will go along with us and counsel patience if they think we have a plan, even a very long-range plan. Our problem, of course, is that we do not have that.[12]

The notion of a plan or strategy became a central requirement if the President was to have a coherent framework for his health message. A bold departure in health care was needed: a proposal that would stake out a unique position for the Administration, based on a clear concept of underlying health system problems. So far, this bold departure had eluded the Administration.

It was early February 1970. The date for the Presidential health message had been set to coincide with the Medicare and Medicaid executive sessions of the Ways and Means Committee to be held late in March. And still, the President had no health message to present to the American people.

---

11. Arthur Hess, memorandum on health care financing options, Deputy Commissioner of the Social Security Administration, Feb. 4, 1970.
12. Lewis H. Butler, memorandum to Arthur Hess, from the Assistant Secretary for Planning and Evaluation, HEW, Feb. 6, 1970.

CHAPTER 2

The Health Maintenance Strategy

Toward the end of 1969, Paul M. Ellwood Jr., M.D., executive director of the American Rehabilitation Foundation (ARF), the Minneapolis-based research arm of the Sister Kenney Institute, was concluding a comprehensive review of the health system and possible ways to reform it, when he made one more of his periodic efforts to bring his ideas to the attention of national health policy leadership.[1] This time, however, his search for policymakers willing to listen coincided with the almost frantic efforts of the Nixon Administration's health leadership to design a coherent national health policy. This time Ellwood's timing was nearly perfect. New public policies often emerge from such chance concurrences.

While the precise time and place for an encounter with top Nixon Administration leadership could not have been plotted or predicted in early 1969, there was little doubt that Ellwood eagerly sought such an encounter. He had tried to get senior health officials of the Johnson Administration to listen to his prescriptions for health system reform without much success. The success that would come in 1970 had been five years in the making.

---

1. The American Rehabilitation Foundation has undergone a number of name changes over the past 10 years. In 1968, the Institute of Interdisciplinary Studies was established within the foundation. It subsequently achieved independent status and, in 1973, the organization's name was shortened to the present InterStudy.

The Origins of Health Maintenance

In 1965, Ellwood, then newly appointed as ARF's executive director, began to reflect on a basic paradox surrounding the foundation's work in rehabilitation medicine: as the Sister Kenney Institute's rehabilitation program improved, utilization and occupancy levels at the Sister Kenney Institute Rehabilitation Hospital began to fall, reducing revenues needed to finance the entire Sister Kenney program. In essence, the best professional efforts of the institute's rehabilitation programs would propel patients out of the hospital's inpatient units into programs of therapy best handled on an outpatient basis. The prevailing system of (inpatient) hospital reimbursement insurance, however, rewarded behavior that was at fundamental odds with the objective of rehabilitation: to make patients mobile and self-reliant. Ellwood was faced with both a practical and moral dilemma. How could the Sister Kenney Institute continue its "good works" when the very success of those efforts would ultimately lead to bankruptcy?

Ellwood's dilemma forced him to search for alternative ways to organize the Sister Kenney Institute, an inquiry that led inevitably to a general analysis and critique of the American health care system. Robert A. Levine's seminal article "Rethinking Our Social Strategies," published in the winter 1968 issue of *The Public Interest,* provided a critical conceptual linkage. Levine had concluded that highly administered social programs "have either not worked, or have worked only on a scale which was very small compared to the size of the problem."[2] Levine would later expand this observation into a full-scale theory of social planning:

> . . . the evidence from both domestic and military systems is clearly consistent with the theory that highly administered and planned systems fail with a high probability. . . . Increasingly, . . . economists . . . have . . . turned to the market system that characterizes our American economy for the answer to many problems. . . . The market business system of the U.S. economy contrasts with a highly administered system because it (1) is decentralized; (2) is self-administered in the sense that most of the prime actors make their own decisions; (3) is motivated by the economic self-interest of these prime actors; (4) requires only the gross application of public policy rather than detailed case-by-case application; (5) is unplanned in the sense of being laid out in advance by external authority.[3]

---

2. Robert A. Levine. Rethinking our social strategies. *Public Interest.* No. 10, winter 1968, p. 88.
3. Robert A. Levine. *Public Planning: Failure and Redirection.* New York City: Basic

Levine recognized the limited capacity of democratic governments in capitalist societies to control the behavior of diverse private markets. He concluded that governmental action worked better where it consciously identified and manipulated incentive structures affecting the behavior of those private markets rather than bypassing them through directly administered bureaucracies. In essence, government ought to expand its reliance on fiscal and monetary policies that make substantial use of private markets, in place of policies requiring complex programs of public management and bureaucratic rule making.

Ellwood and his associates synthesized their own experiences in rehabilitation medicine with Levine's observations into a general systems analysis called "structural incentive analysis." It was based on the principle that social system behavior was responsive to the incentives and rewards of surrounding environments.[4] Thus, health care systems were misbehaving because their component parts were rewarded for such misbehavior.

Structural incentive analysis clearly disclosed that the federal government's so-called solutions to health system problems were really only symptom-directed palliatives. The Comprehensive Health Planning program of the late 1960s, for example, predictably would have failed, according to structural incentive analysis, because it did not alter the underlying incentive structures of health systems. The need to control the overproduction of hospital beds would be subverted by those interests that required continued and expanded use of beds for income or medical research. Only the most disciplined regulatory program might work — certainly not a program based on the voluntary compliance of institutions whose interests were contrary to planning objectives.

Similarly, Medicare and Medicaid would rapidly accelerate inflationary pressures by supplying health systems with virtually unlimited dollars to pay for expanded population coverage. But the health resources were not available in sufficient amounts and in appropriate

---

Books, Inc. 1972, p. 19. See also: Charles L. Schultze. *The Public Use of Private Interest.* Washington, DC: The Brookings Institution, 1977. Both Levine and Schultze argue forcefully in favor of market systems because they create multiple organizational channels to accomplish their purposes. The lack of competition in public bureaucracies is considered to be a major cause of ineffective public programs. A partial solution to this problem is the deliberate creation of competing bureaus to accomplish similar tasks.

4. This approach had been used intuitively by ARF for several years. It was later explicitly recognized as a powerful systematic analytic tool and formalized by Walter McClure, who coined the name. A recent description is given in: Walter McClure. The medical care system under national health insurance: four models. *J. Health Politics, Policy, and Law.* 1:22-68, spring 1976.

locations and practice mixes to absorb these expanded entitlements. Thus, while solving the accessibility problems of the elderly and the poor, on one level, Medicare and Medicaid would drive up the costs of delivering care to all population sectors. And just over the horizon was national health insurance, which, unless implemented in a sophisticated manner, would further exacerbate inflation.

Ellwood and his colleagues had been considering the health care corporation concept since mid-1967 as the most logical comprehensive mechanism to alter the perverse incentives surrounding health care financing. As public and private revenues for the purchase of health services continued to grow, the need for more efficient delivery system organizations became especially critical. Only through such disciplined organizations could the health system find the means to balance the flow of revenue to purchase health services with a sufficient array of health service resources. The two most frequently cited examples of organized health care delivery systems were prepaid group practice plans and foundations for medical care. Ellwood and his associates came to regard these vital, if largely ignored, variations in American medical care organization as the principal ingredients of any serious health care reform proposals. They were, in fact, drawing upon a long history in the evolution of alternative forms of medical practice. The three most significant milestones were: the development of group practices of medicine, the wedding of prepayment to the group practice concept, and the more recent (reactive) development of foundations for medical care.

* * *

The idea of groups of physicians organizing to provide comprehensive health care to patients is as old as the Republic. It is a response to the basic need to provide access to care for defined populations. The Boston Dispensary, founded in 1770, represented an early example of group-based medical care offered to that city's poor. Group medical practice was not considered as a serious alternative to conventional solo practice for the mainstream of the population until 1883, when the Mayo Clinic was founded in Rochester, Minnesota. The success of the Mayo brothers led to the formation of medical groups in other large cities. By 1969, the American Medical Association reported that 6,371 medical groups were actively engaged in practice.

The modern movement of prepaid group practice plans can be traced to the formation, in 1929, of the Ross-Loos Clinic in Los Angeles and to the Elk City Cooperative in Elk City, Oklahoma.[5] The Ross-Loos plan organized a group practice of physicians to contract, on a prepaid basis, for the care of workers in the city's water department. The success of Ross-Loos fomented a long battle between the local medical society and the clinic, because solo practice physicians feared the economic challenge of what derisively came to be called "contract medicine."

If the Ross-Loos experience represented a challenge from within the medical profession, the Elk City Cooperative presented an even more dire threat: consumer-controlled health care plans. The years of the Depression were particularly harsh for rural Americans, and the success of the Elk City Cooperative offered real hope to farm communities for a chance to receive high-quality health care at modest costs. Here, too, organized medicine reacted with alarm to an alien threat. For 20 years, 1934 to 1954, the Elk City Cooperative fought a continuous war with the county and state medical societies of Oklahoma, which threw every possible obstacle in the way of the plan. The threat to organized medicine lay in the consumer control of the plan through the shareholder arrangement, the fixed-sum prepayment, disengaging the level of service from amount of compensation (that is, the fee), and the salaried basis of the physicians employed by the plan. The Elk City Cooperative's medical staff was ousted from the local medical society, and this tactic was applied to other medical groups across the nation. Attempts were made, in many instances, to revoke the licenses of group practice physicians to practice medicine. In virtually all cases, court decisions favored the group physicians, freeing them from further harassment by their fee-for-service colleagues.

Organized medicine clearly favored the voluntary insurance plans, Blue Cross-Blue Shield, and their for-profit competitors, the indemnity insurance companies, as effective ways to counter the consumer-controlled cooperative health care movement. What is most striking about the evolution of these twin forces in medical care organization is their politics: the Blues and indemnity plans were the health industry's response to the economic crisis of the 1930s, and they established the kind of financing arrangements preferred by providers; the cooperative movement, conversely, was the consumer's response to the crisis in health care precipitated by the Depression.

Prior to 1932, the dominant mode of financing medical care services was the patient making direct payment of fees for services rendered. Fee-

---

5. See: William A. MacColl, M.D. *Group Practice & Prepayment of Medical Care*, Washington, DC: Public Affairs Press, 1966, for an excellent review of the historical evolution of the prepaid group practice of medicine.

for-service reimbursement applied equally to physicians and hospitals. Despite its merit in protecting professional autonomy, the fee-for-service system became a highly unreliable source of revenue during the Depression; all the more so, as the health system was in the process of transition from independent professionals to institutionalized and specialized units that required large and stable revenues in order to operate. Some way had to be found to reduce the uncertainties of cash flows inherent in the irregularity of fee-for-service payment. Prepayment provided the answer.

Thus, in 1932, the American Hospital Association responded to the problem of shrinking revenues by adopting an interesting experiment begun in 1929 by a group of school teachers in Dallas, Texas, who had entered into an arrangement with Baylor Hospital for the provision of hospital room and board and specified ancillary services at a predetermined monthly rate. From this emerged Blue Cross, the first modern health insurance plan. The objective of Blue Cross was to reduce the dependence of hospitals on the erratic behavior and fragile finances of patients. Blue Cross would operate as a fiscal intermediary between patients (subscribers) and hospitals, collecting fixed premiums for specified hospital benefits and reimbursing hospitals on the basis of incurred costs.

Blue Cross-Blue Shield offered an attractive way to solve critical economic problems without disrupting established patterns of medical care organization favored by most physicians and hospitals. The Blue Cross-American Hospital Association concept of prepayment helped hospitals attain a degree of stability in their cash flows. Blue Cross did not propose to dictate allowable charges. Increased costs were simply passed on to consumers in higher premium rates, deductibles, and/or copayments. It is not surprising, therefore, that in the late 1930s hospitals and organized medicine eagerly embraced Blue Cross plans and Blue Shield as reforms that could block a drive for more revolutionary changes in medical care organization. For the heart of the consumer-sponsored, cooperative health care plans was the assignment of economic risk to providers and hospitals. By providing an institutional framework within which groups of physicians would offer services under prospectively agreed upon, fixed price contracts, the providers of health care were, in effect, put at direct economic risk for their practice patterns and health care management decisions.

In 1937, the consumer cooperative movement established its first foothold in a large, urban setting with the formation of the Group Health Association (GHA) in Washington, DC. The immediate idea for GHA's incorporation came from employees of the Homeowners Loan Corporation, an agency of the federal government, that sought to lessen the rate of mortgage defaults by reducing the impact of catastrophic illness, the most common source of foreclosures.

Other components of the health consumer community soon began to take responsibility for health care services. An industrial base was established for the cooperative movement with the entry of Kaiser Industries into the health care delivery picture. Sidney Garfield, M.D., and his associates had organized a group practice to serve the needs of construction workers on canal projects crossing the Southern California desert from the Colorado River to the agricultural and metropolitan areas. When the Kaiser organization began the Grand Coulee Dam Project in the state of Washington, Garfield was called upon to establish a prepaid group practice mechanism for Kaiser employees and their families that would offer them workmen's compensation coverage as well as general hospital and medical care.

The Grand Coulee experience was replicated by Kaiser Industries in other areas of the West Coast during World War II, as its industrial activities expanded and work force increased. A new corporate structure, the Permanente Foundation, was formed to manage the evolving prepaid health care system. After the war, the program was opened to the general public and the organizational forms that would carry the program forward to the present were established. Three basic components to the Kaiser Foundation Medical Care Program were introduced. Kaiser Foundation Health Plan, Inc., the enrollment arm of the program, issues medical and hospital service contracts to the general public. The contracts bind the Health Plan to provide required hospital and medical services. To do so, the Health Plan contracts with one of the independent Permanente Medical Groups, organized to serve a particular geographic area. Similarly, the Health Plan contracts with Kaiser Foundation Hospitals for covered hospital services.

These early experiences in prepaid health care demonstrated the viability and flexibility of the concept. The movement spread from rural to urban areas and industrial settings. By the late 1940s, a vigorous minority movement in medical care organization was in full swing: New York City established the Health Insurance Plan of Greater New York (HIP) in 1944, Community Health Center of Two Harbors, Minnesota, also opened its doors in 1944; Rip Van Winkle Clinic, serving the upper Hudson River Valley of New York state, was established in 1946; and Group Health Cooperative of Puget Sound was established in 1947.

A major development, at least from a political standpoint, was the entry of labor unions into the movement: the Teamsters established the Labor Health Institute of St. Louis in 1945; in 1946, the United Mine Workers Welfare and Retirement Fund began to investigate the quality of health care services in the mining regions of Appalachia and was ultimately impelled to establish a chain of hospitals and group medical practices throughout the region; in 1956, the United Auto Workers established the Community Health Association in Detroit.

A forecast of more recent interest in prepaid plans by commercial insurance firms came about in 1956 when the St. Paul-based Group Health Mutual Insurance Company broke with tradition and offered direct, prepaid health services under the Group Health Plan, Inc. The unique sponsorship of this plan indicated the possibility of building insurance industry interest in this approach. Indemnity plans were not the only, nor necessarily the best, way to ensure the availability of health care services.

Throughout the 1930s and 1940s, the development of prepaid group practice was greeted by steady resistance from the ranks of fee-for-service medicine. By 1971, 22 states had enacted laws, usually at the behest of their state and county medical societies, prohibiting the establishment of organizations to engage in "corporate medical practice, conjointly with nonphysicians." Many court challenges were undertaken by consumer groups supporting prepaid group practice formation, and, in most cases, the courts vindicated the incipient consumer plans.

A more positive reaction, however, came from some physicians, who, while viewing prepaid group practice as a threat to their mode of practice, chose to fight back, not by harassing their fellow physicians, but by developing their own innovative medical care organization. Just as the Depression simultaneously spawned the voluntary health insurance programs and prepaid groups, so the threat of prepaid group plans led directly to the birth of a countermovement within fee-for-service medicine: foundations for medical care (FMCs).

By 1954, the Kaiser Foundation Health Plans had become well-established, rapidly spreading their public enrollments up and down the West Coast. Labor organizations in the San Joaquin Valley, dissatisfied with the medical care available to their constituents, began to discuss the establishment of yet another Kaiser-affiliated prepaid group. Local fee-for-service solo practitioners, threatened as in other parts of the country, expressed their concern to the County Medical Society. The result was a decision to apply a collective corporate solution to the challenge by borrowing a page from the Kaiser organization. The local physicians sponsored an independent, nonprofit foundation to address underlying problems in the medical care services available to the community.

At the core of the San Joaquin experiment was the desire to preserve the professional autonomy of fee-for-service medicine while providing an organizational framework to limit costs and improve the quality of care. In one sense, the challenge facing FMC planners was even greater than that facing their group practice counterparts: to harmonize the cost-efficient features of prepayment with the professional autonomy associated with fee-for-service medical practice.

The San Joaquin planners established a prepaid health insurance program that included a minimum package of ambulatory and hospital benefits based on a careful analysis of the needs of the local community. The foundation then contracted with Blue Cross to serve as fiscal intermediary for the established benefit package. Next, the foundation adopted the California relative value study (CRVS) and local conversion factors as the sole basis for establishing fee schedules for each provided service. All community physicians who chose to participate as members of the FMC had to agree to accept these fee schedules and also to accept payments according to the relative value system. Finally, a peer review system was instituted to determine the appropriateness of physicians' practice patterns:

> It is obvious that in setting up a prepaid health-service activity, some type of control of payment to physicians is necessary, and since the comprehensive FMC is dedicated to the fee-for-service principle of reimbursement, no program can be actuarially sound without agreement by physicians on maximum fees coupled with appropriate peer review to prevent overutilization of treatments and procedures.[6]

As experience with the plan accumulated, physicians began to adjust their service patterns according to peer review criteria and their fees were adjusted by reference to the fixed-sum, prepayment pool of dollars collected as insurance premiums. In the early years of some foundations' experiences, fees were sometimes paid at reduced rates to keep the insurance pool solvent. More often, however, the experience has been just the opposite: a moderate portion of the underwriting risk has been distributed to physicians as a bonus — provided, of course, that an "at-risk" program has been established as part of the FMC's basic design. In this setting, physician members accept the risk of losses as well as the bonuses of efficiency.

---

6. Richard H. Egdahl, M.D. Foundations for medical care. *New Engl. J. Med.* 288:491, Mar. 8, 1973, p. 492.

These are the basic elements of the comprehensive FMC whose prototype is the San Joaquin FMC. "In contrast to the comprehensive FMC, the claim-review FMC does not design and sponsor prepaid health programs or set minimum benefits of coverage."[7] The peer review program, typical of both types of FMC, provided the prototype for the federal government's Professional Standards Review Organization (PSRO) program.

The FMC model of medical care organization has been criticized from both the liberal and conservative wings of the health care system. Conservatives, led by the American Medical Association, have generally been less than enthusiastic. It has tended to regard the FMC as a slightly less obnoxious form of prepaid group practice, albeit one without a closed panel and single facility. The AMA fears that it is impossible "to preserve a true fee-for-service system within the framework of a capitation payment in which fixed dollars are available for comprehensive health services."[8] Proponents counter that these fears are largely unfounded:

> There seems to be no reason why a planned comprehensive health program involving known utilization patterns and agreement on the use of fee schedules could not develop reasonably accurate figures for capitation payments for the area's population. Indeed, a combination of careful scrutiny of utilization patterns, vigorous peer review, agreement on fee schedules, and maximum use of health-care technology and allied health personnel appears to be the basic mechanism through which it will be possible to regain control of presently runaway health-care costs.[9]

At the other extreme, proponents of prepaid group practice argue that the FMC structure is too loose and, therefore, shares many of the inefficiencies of an unorganized delivery system. Since 1959, however, when certain FMCs were qualified as carriers by the Federal Employees Health Benefits Program (FEHBP), under the new terminology "individual practice associations (IPAs)," a comparative data base has been established to answer many of these questions. The evidence augurs reasonably well for FMCs. Comparisons among the three general types of qualified FEHBP plans — Blue Cross-Blue Shield service benefit plans, indemnity insurance plans, and prepaid group practice plans/IPAs

---

7. Richard H. Egdahl, M.D., *Ibid.*, p. 492.
8. Ernest B. Howard, M.D., executive vice-president, American Medical Association, quoted in *Medical World News*, Dec. 3, 1971.
9. Richard H. Egdahl, M.D., *op. cit.*, p. 492.

— on hospital utilization rates, disclose that the few FMCs (or IPAs) qualified by FEHBP keep patient days well below the service benefit and indemnity plans and only slightly higher than prepaid groups. Premium costs have also been comparable to the groups and well below indemnity plan premiums.

In short, a few of the strongly structured FMCs, over the past 20 years, have proven their viability and durability as cost-efficient innovations in medical care organization. Along with prepaid groups, they could offer real opportunities for innovation on a broad national scale.

* * *

These evolutionary developments in health care organization and financing were essentially private sector responses to the changing fortunes of medicine during a period of rapid scientific progress and dramatic economic upheaval. The twin pressures of scientific progress and economic depression lent urgency and pace to the various movements and countermovements of the 1930s and 1940s.

The federal government was not absent from nor indifferent to these evolving trends. Prior to 1935, the federal government played a relatively restricted role in financing personal health care services. Public health functions were virtually limited to areas of collective service, such as communicable disease control programs, milk and water supply, inspection of food handlers, and so forth.

A minimal federal role in personal health services had been established early, by the 5th Congress, which created the Marine Hospital Service in 1798. Emerging later as the U.S. Public Health Service, this agency took a major role in collecting and disseminating health statistics and in providing direct health services to designated wards of the federal government, particularly the military and native American populations, that is, Indians, Eskimos, and Aleuts.

The delivery of personal medical services to the bulk of the population was held to be a private, not a public, enterprise. In 1935, however, the Social Security Act authorized federal grants-in-aid to the states for general public health programs and maternal and child health care. About the same time, the Farm Security Administration began to build health care programs for rural areas, and, during World War II, a program for emergency maternity and infant care (EMIC) was established for the dependents of servicemen. The principle of direct federal support for delivery of health services to poverty populations and to wards of the government had thus become firmly established.

These limited forays into the realm of health services delivery had been effectively slowed by the pressures of World War II and the increasing tendency toward substantial federal subsidy of medical science and technology. Beginning in 1936, with the National Cancer Act, and accelerating dramatically after the War, Congress committed the federal government to an all-out assault on the "dread diseases," through basic and applied medical research. The growth of these investments has been substantial. In 1946, the federal government inaugurated the Hill-Burton Health Facilities Construction program. Over the years, in no small measure because of the ready availability of federal funding, the supply of hospital beds has increased to the point where the United States is considered to be oversupplied by a factor of 25 percent to 33 percent.

A primary effect of federal investment policies in health between 1940 and 1975 has been to sharpen the focus on hospital-based care, specialization, and scientific achievement. These trends have helped to increase the costs of delivering medical care by concentrating service in expensive institutional settings, encouraging utilization of costly medical technologies, and fragmenting health care delivery among many quasi-autonomous producers (specialists who, for the most part, continue to price and charge for their work on a piecework, fee-for-service basis).

Federal programs have attacked the problems of cost and availability from differing vantage points, employing various fiscal and economic mechanisms. The Kerr-Mills program and its replacement, Medicaid, subsidized payment for a broad range of services to entitled populations. Medicare, likewise, subsidized the demand side of the health care economy. It was not a welfare program, but it was administered centrally by the federal government and offered comprehensive health services to elderly citizens.

Project grant programs were administered directly by the federal health bureaucracies and their locally based institutional clients. In the early years, administrators did very little to coordinate the vendor payments that augmented consumer purchasing power with the projects augmenting available health resources. For example, in many cases, neighborhood health centers, already fully funded under federal grants, failed to recover Medicare and Medicaid reimbursements on patients who had such coverage. In effect, public subsidies were wasted through such double coverage.

In general, federal policies governing the health system have been poorly planned and coordinated. Programs established to solve one set of problems created new ones. Policies established under particular historical circumstances lingered beyond their usefulness. Resource development subsidies designed to stimulate expansion of health facilities became a major cause of overproduction of hospital beds and maldistribution of advanced technology. Biomedical research and training grants promoted excessive proliferation of medical specialties and obstructed development of community-based general medical practice. Third-party payments reimbursing hospital and specialized medical services tended to bloat medicine's pricing structure, to eliminate consumer choice from the purchasing process, while exaggerating the real need for these services. Meanwhile, services actually most needed by people (general and family medicine) became progressively more scarce as various federal policies supported the trend toward specialization and high-cost technology. Governmental subsidies, in short, have magnified and intensified the health system's internal contradictions.

Medicare and Medicaid investments stimulated demand for without providing significant expansions in the supply of primary and community-based services. The inevitable strain on already maldistributed medical care resources fueled the massive inflation that, by early 1969, led to a frantic search for corrective policies. This search for national health policy became the principle preoccupation of the federal health establishment, just as Paul Ellwood began to promote the virtues of health care corporations.

From Concept to National Health Policy

The health care corporation idea (the prototypes of which were prepaid group practices and FMCs) was the primary item on Ellwood's agenda in meetings with top Public Health Service officials during 1969. Significantly, Ellwood was appointed to a special advisory group to then Assistant Secretary for Health and Scientific Affairs Roger Egeberg, M.D., and served on a scientific and professional advisory board to Paul J. Sanazaro, M.D., then director of the National Center for Health Services Research and Development (NCHSRD). In December 1969, Ellwood presented the health care corporation idea as the key structural reform required by health care delivery systems. Egeberg seemed sympathetic to the idea, but took no concrete action to promote it within HEW. Neither did Sanazaro.

Prepaid groups and FMCs were no strangers to the federal health bureaucracies. In fact, Ellwood's proposal for vigorous federal promotion of prepaid health plans was met with indifference by the Public

Health Service primarily because developmental efforts were already proceeding on a limited scale. Ellwood, it seems, had not offered the health bureaucracies any new information. Nor was the Public Health Service in a position to respond to the notion that prepaid health care should become the central focus of national health policy. The Public Health Service, Ellwood soon learned, was not the place where health policies were made; rather, it was where health programs to implement established policies were executed.

To be sure, the Medicare and Medicaid amendments (Title XVIII and XIX of the Social Security Act) provided for experimentation with incentive reimbursement; although, as of 1969, only one prepaid plan, the Health Insurance Plan of New York (HIP), had successfully negotiated a prospective reimbursement arrangement under the Medicare program. Moreover, while the potential for utilization of Medicaid as a lever to develop optional plans of prepaid health care for the poor had not gone unnoticed by the Medical Services Administration, its parent agency, the Social and Rehabilitation Services (SRS), had failed to promulgate regulations governing state participation in prepayment plans. This failure acted as a powerful disincentive for states to enter into such innovative Title XIX arrangements.

The Medical Care Administration of the Public Health Service had established a health economics branch in 1962 with a strong intellectual commitment to prepaid health care plans, group practice plans in particular. In 1968, the Office of Group Practice Development was established. This office began, on a limited basis, to provide seed money contracts and grants for the development of prepaid plans. A small planning contract was awarded to the Group Health Association of America (GHAA) in 1967 for the purpose of organizing a labor union-oriented prepaid group practice plan. GHAA was awarded an additional $5 million grant in 1969 to develop prepaid group practices in some 33 cities. The project did not accomplish this objective, although it served as a useful guide as to what should and should not be done in trying to establish prepaid plans.

These limited developmental efforts were highly fragmented and clearly not part of a coordinated national health strategy. Moreover, the Bureau of Health Insurance (BHI), which administered Medicare, exhibited no great enthusiasm for prepayment. Indeed, BHI lent only limited encouragement to negotiations for prospective reimbursement contracts with prepaid plans under existing legislative authority.

In short, while the permanent health bureaucracies could literally respond to Ellwood's presentation with the claim that "we are already doing it," that response was exaggerated. The health bureaucracies, in 1969, were pursuing prepaid health care in a limited and uncoordinated manner. And, most assuredly, they ignored the potentialities of prepayment as a tool both for developing leverage over a health care system badly in need of reorganization and for maximizing federal investments in health within a coherent health fiscal policy. These policy matters seemed to be beyond the grasp and concern of the technocrats in the permanent health bureaucracies.

Underlying this lack of interest in prepaid health plans was the simple fact that this mode of medical care programming was not, after all, central to prescribed federal activities in the health care field. Medicare had been established as a cost-reimbursing social insurance program paralleling the structure of Blue Cross-Blue Shield and commercial health insurance plans. Medicaid was actually a state-administered federal grant program, which reimbursed the costs of certain types and amounts of health care for welfare-eligible segments of the population. Neither program sought to reshape health care systems. Indeed, Medicare administrators were expressly precluded from doing so by Section 1801 of the Social Security Act.

The health agencies of HEW, although not openly hostile to prepaid health care, were only marginally interested in it. They were ready to devote some demonstration monies to the idea, but not on a scale that would appear to challenge their primary commitment to reimbursement of incurred costs and categorical project grant programs.

Not until Ellwood made contact with the most senior HEW officials, themselves struggling with the health crisis, did he begin to make headway with his ideas for health care reform. The opportunity came in February 1970, when a significant milestone was reached in the search for national health policy.

* * *

Major public policies, like scientific breakthroughs, often result from the efforts of many individuals and the coincidence of small, sometimes hardly noticed, events and decisions. The threshold of significant occurrences in science and public policy, however, can often be traced to a moment of discovery. There is the precise moment the microbiologist isolates an elusive virus strain or the critical meeting when policymakers n array of conceptual and political strands into a coherent statement of policy. Just such a critical meeting occurred in Washington, DC, during the afternoon and evening of Thursday, February 5, 1970. It was an important event, both in terms of the ideas that emerged and as a case study of how major new policies sometimes find their way onto the nation's health policy agenda.

The meeting provided an opportunity for a small group of people to assemble old facts and old ideas into a framework that yielded a new idea: health maintenance organizations. Although the concepts and elements of health maintenance organizations existed long before February 5, 1970, only thereafter did they fit into a configuration of organizational forms that were collectively labeled HMOs. Before that date, there were only health care corporations, prepaid group practices, individual (foundation) practice associations, neighborhood health centers, and clinics; after February 5, each of these organizational forms were seen as sharing features common to all HMOs, yet maintaining certain unique features as well.

The meeting was held in Washington, DC, in Ellwood's Dupont Plaza Hotel room. Ellwood was hosting the meeting at the request of Tom Joe, Under Secretary John G. Veneman's special assistant at HEW. Besides Ellwood and Joe, the meeting was attended by Veneman, Assistant Secretary for Planning and Evaluation Lewis Butler, and Thomas Georges, M.D., a professor of community medicine from Temple University. The meeting began late on that Thursday afternoon and lasted into the early hours of Friday morning. Butler, Veneman, and Joe had come to engage in a general discussion with Ellwood on possible approaches the Administration could take to control the costs of the Medicare and Medicaid programs. Joe's previous contacts with Ellwood had led him to believe that something useful could emerge from such a meeting. Georges had been invited by Joe as a professional observer; or, more bluntly stated, Georges was there to verify for the nonphysicians present that Ellwood's presentation made sense from a health and medical care point of view. They could judge for themselves the political and economic usefulness of his proposals.

The meeting began with Ellwood, Joe, Veneman, and Georges present. Butler was to arrive later. Veneman opened by restating briefly the government's basic problem: how to deal with the cost overruns in the Medicare and Medicaid programs. He then turned the discussion over to Ellwood, who opened by making three points. First, the problems of inflation and resource maldistribution would not be solved by continued federal tinkering with narrow aspects of the health system or by more regulatory control. Present federal interventions in the health system merely exacerbated the observed distortions that produced inflation. Ellwood's second point was that the full range of federal economic, legal, and persuasive power had to be coordinated in an effort to restructure the health care delivery system. His final point was that some means had to be found to develop precise future directions for the health care delivery system. It would not be enough to leave the details up to voluntary and cooperative planning efforts such as Comprehensive Health Planning and Regional Medical Programs.

Underlying these ideas was the basic premise of structural incentive analysis: that the health system was behaving according to the incentives placed in and around it. If the performance of the health system fell short on various efficiency and equity criteria, it was because the individual products of each one of the system's components did not add up to an acceptable overall product. It might be sensible, for example, for a hospital to seek more efficient ways to keep its beds filled, in order to maintain appropriate revenues, even though the success of that policy would yield even more inflation in overall health care costs. Therefore, the federal government should examine the full range of incentives motivating health system behavior and try to modify those incentives that promote dysfunctional behavior. This analysis led Ellwood to observe that the present health system treated people almost exclusively when they were sick, relying extensively on expensive curative medical care, and that incentives to provide less expensive, ambulatory, preventive, and early diagnostic services were generally lacking.

No sooner had Ellwood presented his analysis of the structural disincentives to efficient health system behavior than Veneman stated, "We buy that. What's your plan?" To Ellwood, this frank acceptance of the idea that incentives could decisively shape health system behavior and the unquestioning recognition that federal policies had promoted perverse incentives signalled the possibility of achieving a major turnaround in federal health policy. No policymaker at the level represented by Veneman had ever before accepted these ideas so readily.

Veneman had long since independently arrived at an analysis of the health system similar to Ellwood's. His seven years in the California Assembly as chairman of the Welfare Committee had not only thoroughly familiarized him with the problems of Medicaid, but had also shown him that

> with the whole health subject and particularly on the provider's side, . . . the incentive is always on the wrong end. If a person gets sick, then, of course, the doctor gets paid. If the guy's in the hospital and the doctor wants to take the weekend off, for example, and goes in and looks at his patient on Friday afternoon and says, well, its kind of a close call, he'll say . . . I'll take off and leave the patient here until Monday and then I'll take a look.[10]

Ellwood proceeded to outline his proposal for correcting these negative incentives and required structural alterations. He proposed that the federal government actively sponsor the formation of health care corporations that would take responsibility for providing comprehensive health care to consumers. As part of a federal strategy to encourage the establishment of these organizations, the government should do four things: prepay, through Medicare and Medicaid, fixed-price contracts for eligible consumers for a combination of inpatient and outpatient medical care; encourage some structural changes, through the formation of group practice prepayment plans; establish enrollment requirements whereby customers would be committed to these health care organizations for a fixed period of time; and ensure quality of care through expanded consumer choice.

Veneman liked the proposal. As a California lawmaker, he was familiar with the prototype health care organizations described by Ellwood — the Kaiser-Permanente Plan and the San Joaquin County Foundation for Medical Care, both California products. That the three top leaders of HEW — Secretary Robert Finch, Veneman, and Butler — were Californians was a coincidence not lost on Ellwood. Moreover, Veneman was already on record, at his July 10 news conference, as favoring federal encouragement of prepayment and incentive reimbursement under Medicare and Medicaid.

Ellwood supplied the conceptual linkages connecting a health fiscal strategy (prepayment) to delivery system structures that would accomplish the government's objective to improve cost-efficiency in its major health care programs. He suggested that the federal government promote formation of health care corporations by making it possible and attractive to use Medicare and Medicaid funds to reimburse these plans on a firm, fixed-price, prospective basis. The financial leverage of federal programs would thus be harnessed to effect structural changes in health care delivery systems. And available data from Kaiser and other prepay-

10. John G. Veneman, interview, Nov. 1973.

ment plans suggested that costs of care under prepayment plans would be less than the costs of care offered on the traditional fee-for-service basis.

Butler joined the group in the evening. By this time, the general strategy presented by Ellwood had been favorably received by Veneman, Georges, and Joe. Veneman charged the group to go forward and work out the details and then left. The discussion then turned to how specifically the evolving strategy might be implemented.

Butler offered an important conceptual alteration to Ellwood's framework. Ellwood had come to the meeting committed to the notion that the government had to use its fiscal authority to promote a particular model of health care organization, group practice prepayment plans, which dictated a precise specification of structure, based essentially on the Kaiser experience. Therefore, as Butler probed for specifics, Ellwood began to detail his views on how many doctors were needed, the number of enrolled consumers, relationships with hospitals, benefit packages, and other specific delivery system arrangements. Butler then inquired, "Are you sure that you've got to encourage group practice or some specific delivery arrangements?"

This led to a discussion of how far the federal government ought to go in specifying new forms of health care organization. Butler had little confidence in the wisdom of government telling people how to do something, rather, he believed that the federal government ought to tell the health system what it wanted done, but not how to do it:

> You never tell people how to do something; tell them what to do and they'll amaze you with their ingenuity. Why should we specify how to put it together? Let the doctors — let everybody do it, figure out how to put it together. Let's specify what we want it to do. And we don't give a damn how they put it together. They can make it a partnership, a corporation, they can make it one of 55 different organizational forms. Let's describe the thing by what we want it to do, not how it's formed.[11]

That was a different idea for Ellwood, which he accepted after only a moment's reflection. The significance of this simple variation on the group practice prepayment theme for the advocacy of the evolving health system reform proposal was profound. By leaving the specification of organizational structures to the delivery system itself but defining incentives designed to accomplish particular objectives, it could be argued that the federal government was removing itself from interference in the direct

---

11. Lewis H. Butler, interview, Nov. 1973.

delivery of health care and confining itself to the role of catalyst and purchaser. The idea could be sold, from this frame of reference, as a market reform strategy rather than yet another federal program requiring a large bureaucracy of civil servants to manage it. This would be exceedingly appealing to a Republican Administration. It would be equally unappealing to a federal health bureaucracy committed to tinkering with small pieces of the delivery system and to the aggrandizement of its own role or to a congressional system of watchdog committees dedicated to tracking very precisely articulated programs involving the spending of federal dollars.

All that would come later. For the moment, it appeared that the Administration had at last found its bold departure in the health arena. But what to call it? The phrase *health maintenance organization* was first used at the February 5 meeting. Ellwood had been toying with the term *health maintenance* while preparing for the meeting. The use of *health* rather than *medical* was desirable, since prevention, early diagnosis, and early treatment was to be emphasized. *Maintenance* focused on maintaining health rather than treating illness. And *organization* was a term possessing a neutrality unavailable in such terms as *corporation, group practice,* or *partnership.* Each of these terms identified a particular medical care structure. The term *health maintenance organization,* however, was unique and not immediately assailable from either the left or the right. It was a politically nebulous and, therefore, desirable phrase. It was also a generic term that precisely conveyed the special nature of the concept taking shape on February 5.[12]

A final component of the health maintenance strategy also emerged on February 5: the ways and means of bringing the concept forward. The initial impetus all along had been the need to control the costs of the Medicare-Medicaid programs. Throughout the late fall and early winter, Veneman had presented testimony on the Administration's welfare reform strategy to the Ways and Means Committee. The committee had been in executive session since the first of the year and was turning to Titles XVIII and XIX in mid-February. If the Administration was to offer proposals beyond those being prepared by HEW, these would have to be presented before executive sessions scheduled to conclude by Tuesday, March 24. Veneman, Butler, and Joe had slightly over six weeks to refine

---

12. Ellwood's coinage of the term *health maintenance organization* was a unique development, although the concept of health maintenance was discussed by Richard Weinerman as early as 1968. See: E. Richard Weinerman. Problems and perspectives of group practice. *Bull. NY Acad. Med.* 44:1423, Nov. 1968.

the health maintenance concept into a legislative proposal that the White House would endorse and, possibly, use as the basis for a Presidential health message. They also had to figure out some way to tie the HMO concept concretely to the fiscal leverage of the Medicare program through an amendment to Title XVIII. Joe suggested a "Part C" amendment, which would add a "prepayment option" to Parts A and B, already enacted.

Butler charged Ellwood with the task of developing a paper "that reflects what we've discussed and come back as fast as you can." He warned Ellwood that although "the future has no call on my time . . . you . . . represent the future, [so] you have to get through."[13]

The basic outline of the health maintenance strategy was in place. Six weeks remained in which to try to reclaim the national health policy initiative for the Nixon Administration. The six weeks that began with the February 5 meeting and concluded with Veneman's March 23 presentation of an HMO option to the House Ways and Means Committee was a period of creative development seldom witnessed in national health affairs. During that time, the health maintenance strategy, initially distilled from an array of health system reform ideas at the Dupont Plaza meeting, was hammered into a full-fledged Administration proposal.

* * *

The setting was opportune. The White House was committed to a Presidential health message to be delivered in late March or early April. Butler was responsible for developing the message and coordinating the work of the informal White House health task force attempting to put it together. Some closure on the matter would have to be reached by March 23, inasmuch as Rep. Wilbur Mills (D-AR) had formally requested that Finch present the Ways and Means Committee with proposals for improving Medicare and Medicaid performance.

The Dupont Plaza meeting had, in fact, occurred against a backdrop of frenetic activity in the HEW Office of the Secretary. Ruth Hanft, Butler's chief health aide, was developing materials for Finch's testimony as well as for the Presidential health message, along with staff from the Social Security Administration, the Medical Services Administration, and the Health Services and Mental Health Administration.[14] HEW's top

---

13. Butler meant that his days were filled with short-term crisis management making it difficult for him to take a long-term view.
14. See chapter 1, pp. 6-11, for a detailed account of this in-house effort.

leadership emerged from the Dupont Plaza meeting hoping that it had found an additional source of analytical input to their health policy development efforts. Ellwood's presentation appeared to offer a refreshingly new and different direction from internally initiated proposals for narrow, incremental changes in Medicare-Medicaid payment mechanisms and tighter regulatory controls.

The health maintenance proposal went through three distinguishable, although overlapping, stages of development between February 5 and March 20: first, the fleshing out of the concept into a national health policy proposal by Ellwood and his staff; second, a restatement of the proposal by Butler, with help from Ellwood and his staff, within the context of the evolving Presidential health message; and the third and final stage, the development of the Part C amendment to Title XVIII of the Social Security Act, the elaboration of this proposal in testimony for the Ways and Means Committee, and the concomitant neutralizing of Social Security Administration and HEW senior staff opposition to the Part C proposal.

Ellwood returned to Minneapolis from his meeting in Washington convinced that, at long last, he had found a sympathetic forum for his ideas on health system reform. Over the next two weeks, he and his staff assembled their thoughts, organized a series of information-gathering field trips, and produced a set of working papers.[15] Butler had not been very explicit, however, as to how the Minneapolis group should structure their written input to the HEW-White House effort. One member of the staff suggested that the health maintenance proposal be couched in the form of a Presidential health message. This meant using simple language and emphasizing the proposal's "impact on people and specified actions to be taken."[16] In short, give the policymakers specific language for the Presidential message.

Nancy Anderson, of Ellwood's staff, drafted an outline, using ideas from the Minneapolis group's working papers, which Ellwood took with him to Washington on Sunday, February 22. He revised this outline, expanded it into a paper, and presented a document entitled "The Health

---

15. Walter McClure took responsibility for developing cost information about HMOs and visited the Social Security Adminstration's Office of Research and Statistics to collect data on various costs of reimbursing extant HMOs compared to fee-for-service systems. Rick Carlson, the lawyer in the group, focused on the problems of legal barriers to starting up HMOs. McClure and Carlson together drafted specifications and legal language for the actual Part C proposal. Nancy Anderson, a sociologist, worked on consumer rights and was the group's writer and synthesizer.

16. Nancy N. Anderson, "Thinking Outline: Health Reform," American Rehabilitation Foundation, Feb. 22, 1970.

Maintenance Plan Health Reform" to Butler on February 25.[17] This paper, written in the language and format of a Presidential message, provided a framework for further ARF input to the HEW health planning process. It convinced Butler that Ellwood and his staff could be of real service. It alerted internal HEW health planners to the fact that Butler and Veneman were receiving organized written input from an outside group. And it marked the end of the actual detailing of the new policy and the beginning of Butler's attempts to place health maintenance on the White House agenda. This would involve selling the new concept to his own HEW staff.

The initial HEW staff response was that while the goals of the health maintenance plan were laudable, "there are real difficulties in getting from where we are now to where the plan wants to go."[18] Certainly, it would not be possible to translate the general goals for developing a health system oriented to health maintenance into a "legislative plan shaping up for the creation of a health maintenance plan."

Opposition to the Minneapolis group's proposal, then, centered around the view that the achievement of the health maintenance plan hinged on the development of a scale of federal intervention that neither the health system nor the government were prepared for. The proposal was too global and ambitious, however commendable its intent, because the mere presence of a prepayment-type reimbursement mechanism would not ensure the development of sufficient numbers of HMOs. Additional subsidies for HMO development would be required. The health maintenance plan did not provide for such subsidies. Was the Administration prepared to undertake a comprehensive effort? Arthur Hess, the deputy commissioner of the Social Security Administration, certainly was not:

> . . . my principal concern is how do you get from where we are now to a "Plan C in Medicare." I think through a process of gradualism along the lines of incentive experiments and the things we have in the Administration's proposal, we have prospects of moving slowly but surely in the directions that are stated to be long-run objectives.[19]

---

17. The February 25, 1970, document restated the underlying principles outlined by Ellwood at the Dupont Plaza meeting and proposed that the federal government should add a Plan C to Medicare, which would offer comprehensive coverage through a prepaid contract with health maintenance organizations. This would require amending Title XVIII (Medicare) of the Social Security Act to enable the elderly to undertake prepaid contracts with appropriate organizations on a permanent basis.
18. Ruth Hanft, "The Health Maintenance Plan," memorandum to the Assistant Secretary for Planning and Evaluation, HEW, Mar. 3, 1970.
19. Arthur E. Hess, "The Health Maintenance Plan," memorandum to Mr. Tom Joe and Mr. Lewis Butler, Social Security Administration, Mar. 2, 1970.

A full-scale, prospective reimbursement alternative that offered a permanent complement to fee-for-service reimbursement was not a welcome prospect.[20]

Butler, however, was sufficiently impressed with the February 25 document to charge Ellwood to prepare "something I could take to the White House."[21] On February 26, Ellwood, now back in Minneapolis, reported to his staff that "Our assignment has lost its ambiguity . . . our job is to develop, over the next eight days, a 'decision paper' on health reform."[22]

The ARF project team organized its work around three areas: the health maintenance contract, the health maintenance organization, and consumer rights and legal and other barriers to implementation. An overview paper was produced, substantially expanding the extended outline of February 25 and entitled "The Health Maintenance Plan." This document was supported by a series of working papers, all of which were organized into a loose-leaf presentation volume, the "Green Book," with "Plan for Health Maintenance System" printed on the cover.[23] About a dozen of the volumes were printed and distributed to a group of HEW health officials, assembled on Saturday morning, March 7, in the HEW Chart Room. The meeting represented the first formal presentation of the health maintenance plan to the HEW health bureaucracy.

The proposal was received unenthusiastically. General reactions at the meeting varied among the participants. There was rather uniform acceptance of the health maintenance plan's objectives but with the caveat that the time was not opportune for this effort. Social Security Administration staff were particularly critical of specific, operational elements of the health maintenance concept. They were concerned about the apparent lack of accountability in the proposal and the emphasis on free-market competition liberally interspersed in the documents Ellwood presented for review.

As one HEW staffer summed up the internal reaction:

---

20. For an excellent discussion of the Social Security Administration's reluctance to embark on innovations that might antagonize providers, see: Judith M. Feder. Social Security and Medicare. In: Kenneth M. Friedman and Stuart H. Rakoff. *Toward a National Health Policy: Public Policy and the Control of Health Care Costs.* Lexington, MA: Lexington Books, 1977, pp. 19-35.
21. Lewis H. Butler, interview, Nov. 1973.
22. Paul M. Ellwood Jr., M.D., "Health Maintenance System Planning," memorandum to staff, American Rehabilitation Foundation, Feb. 26, 1970.
23. Lewis H. Butler, upon seeing the cover emblazoned with "Plan for Health Maintenance System," asked Ellwood to remove "Plan for" and "System" leaving the phrase "Health Maintenance." He had learned that in the skeptical HEW environment, too much dramatization of an innovation could lead to its early demise.

> There ensued an internal fight — Ellwood's definitions were too loose. Many of us challenged his concept of competing HMOs across the street from each other and the whole free market and the waste of resources . . . we were not critical of the concept . . . Ellwood's thinking to a large extent was very sloppy.

Veneman was annoyed that the health bureaucrats would challenge his policy judgments, believing that their role was not to counsel on timing or other "political factors," but solely on the technical merits (or demerits) of the health maintenance proposal. Joe found the bureaucrats' inability to separate technical detail from high policy understandable, but frustrating. Ellwood and his staff were discouraged by their reception and saw the meeting as a Social Security-inspired attack on the health maintenance plan.

The health maintenance planning effort was not halted as a result of the meeting with the health bureaucracies. As Veneman noted:

> I do remember the initial reaction from the Social Security Administration wasn't very favorable . . . and we sort of made it very clear that this wasn't an option on their part . . . the decision had been made . . . and we were going to roll with a Part C.[24]

The health maintenance plan proposed a comprehensive health policy, which, in the long run, would be the global framework for all future health care policies:

> Existing proposals speak to what needs reforming about the health system . . . but . . . tackle one or two problems and thus tend to miss the point that the only possible reform is one which makes the system more self-regulating so that intervention and tinkering will not become increasingly necessary.[25]

The key element in the plan was the endorsement of HMOs by the federal government and the vigorous promotion of this form of medical care delivery under Titles XVIII and XIX through the addition of Part C and other appropriate legislation.

Internal opposition to the proposal continued throughout early March, substantially reflecting the reluctance of the Social Security Administration and senior HEW health planners to embrace the health maintenance plan. Hanft argued:

---

24. John G. Veneman, interview, Nov. 1973.
25. "The Health Maintenance Plan — Health Reform," draft, HEW/Office of the Secretary, Feb. 25, 1970.

> After reading the larger document, my original feelings remain much the same. This is a plan that is from 10 to 20 years in the future unless the Federal government is willing to provide large amounts of front end money to start thousands of these.[26]

Concerning the key elements of a Presidential message endorsing the concept and the Part C proposal, Hanft argued against both. The former would place the Administration:

> in a position where it has endorsed a global plan whose results wouldn't be visible for 10-15-20 years. Building up public expectations without being able to achieve short-range visible results could boomerang.

The health maintenance strategy combined comprehensiveness with simplicity, making it both a source of attractiveness to HEW's senior Republican leadership and of suspicion to top-level career health policy makers. Because HMOs were not merely new kinds of health care organizations, but really alternative, comprehensive health care delivery systems, they offered hope not only for improving health system efficiency, but also for raising the quality of care and the overall health level of the population. Veterans of previous federal ventures into grand health policy designs, however, believed that HMOs and HEW were promising more than they both could deliver.

The tempo of activities increased following the March 7 meeting. Butler worked with the ARF group on Saturday afternoon and on through Sunday, March 8. The "Health Maintenance Plan" document was tightened and refined. An essential new strategic element was to frame the entire package of specific proposals as presenting a choice between promoting "a health maintenance industry that is largely self-regulating" versus reliance on "continued or increased federal intervention through regulation, investment, and planning."[27] This dichotomy dramatized in heightened form the political-ideological attractiveness of the health maintenance plan for the Republican Administration.

According to the Republicans, the health maintenance approach would change the federal role in health affairs to one of providing "investment capital" to stimulate market reform. The previous Democratic Administration had insisted on a much broader role, one that placed ex-

---

26. Ruth S. Hanft, "Health Maintenance Plan," memorandum to Lewis H. Butler, HEW/Office of the Secretary, Mar. 9, 1970.
27. Paul M. Ellwood Jr., and others, "The Health Maintenance Strategy," Mar. 9, 1970.

cessive reliance on regulations, detailed federal planning requirements, and categorical grant-in-aid types of program investments. The federal approaches of the past were themselves major contributors to health system chaos. Rather than representing greater intervention in the health system, as suggested by its critics, the health maintenance plan promised to reduce the federal role in health care.

The "Health Maintenance Plan" paper was finally ready on March 9. Throughout the month of February, Butler had been meeting weekly with the White House health task force and had alerted them generally to the effort he had undertaken with Ellwood. The insertion of the health maintenance plan on the White House agenda, therefore, was not considered to be a dramatic event because Butler had carefully laid the groundwork for the emergence of HMO.

The White House Endorses the Health Maintenance Strategy

Although the informal White House health task force began to discuss possible approaches to a Presidential health message before the Christmas holidays, no specific work was accomplished until the middle of January, and Butler, its chairman, had no substantive proposals available until early February. The results of HEW internal staff work left Butler searching for new insights and approaches to national health policy. Clearly, he was not satisfied with the conventional approaches being offered by his staff.

The complexity of health system problems indicated that a health message offering solutions or even detailing a systematic course of action would be nearly impossible to complete by late March, the agreed upon target date for the President's message. A meeting held with a group of prominent health economists during this period only underscored the confusion of Butler and his colleagues; they were literally awash with a bewildering array of issues and possible courses of action. No one seemed to be able to provide Butler with a structured plan of action. He was frankly worried that the White House work group might not be able to pull together a coherent health policy for the President.

The White House health task force received a copy of the March 9 "Health Maintenance Plan" paper written by Ellwood and the Minneapolis group with understandable expectations. Richard Nathan, one of the task force's members, provided a comprehensive list of reform proposals that had been floating around for the past three months. The health maintenance plan proposal was now added to that list. In effect, the White House health task force, through Nathan's memorandum, gave Butler the green light to go ahead and put a document together that included the health maintenance proposal.[28] On March 18, then, Butler submitted an outline for the Presidential health message. Most significantly, the outline contained an option for HMOs.

Now Butler had to convince his own HEW staff that the health maintenance approach should be the most important component of the forthcoming Presidential message. On Thursday and Friday, March 19 and 20, Butler met almost continuously with his HEW staff on the health message project — Hanft and Hess from HEW; Ellwood and Robert Eilers, a health economist from the University of Pennsylvania, from the outside. Ellwood, of course, was committed to health maintenance, and Butler, having now been exposed to the health maintenance idea for six weeks, was long since convinced that it was the appropriate framework for organizing the health message. His HEW staff was another matter, and, throughout Friday, March 20, there were arguments pro and con, with the staff taking the negative position. Finally, however, Butler affirmed that he was going forward with a health maintenance-oriented message, and his staff acceded to his wishes.

On Saturday, March 21, 1970, Butler sat down in his office to write two papers. One of them was a decision paper to go to the President to be signed by Presidential adviser John Ehrlichman.[29] The other was the message that was to go with the paper.[30] Butler delivered these two papers to the White House later that day.

The memorandum to the President for Ehrlichman's signature laid out the options available to the President. For the short term, the federal government ought to intensify efforts to control federal costs by eliminating "cost plus" hospital reimbursement and by restraining excessive physician fees. For the long term, the government should use its huge federal purchasing power under Medicare and Medicaid to accelerate changes in health care delivery by encouraging the growth of HMOs, which could deliver care at a fixed annual fee. The goal would be to create competitive alternatives to the usual methods for providing health care. Such organizations would have an incentive to control costs and to keep the patient healthy. Specifically, the long-term strategy would require legislative changes authorizing various cost control mechanisms; legislative changes in Medicare to permit annual contracts with HMOs; legislation authorizing statewide experiments under

---

28. Richard P. Nathan, "Listing of Major Health Reform Proposals," memorandum to Lewis H. Butler, and others, OMB, Mar. 10, 1970.
29. Memorandum to the President, unsigned draft, Mar. 21, 1970.
30. "Health Message," unsigned draft, Mar. 21, 1970.

Medicaid for purchase of health care for the poor from such organizations; and, finally, conditioning state Medicaid participation on removing legal barriers to the functioning of such organizations, inasmuch as such barriers then existed in about one-half of the states.

The memorandum then took up arguments in favor of a Presidential health message to present the Administration's strategy to Congress. The President had three choices. He could present a Presidential message announcing these proposals. Or he could issue a short, two- or three-page Presidential endorsement of HEW actions in presenting his proposals. Finally, the President could remain entirely silent on health, leaving Finch to put out any message that was appropriate. This choice, in effect, would delay a major Presidential statement on health until later in 1970, or, more probably, until January 1971. The advantages and disadvantages of each option were discussed.

As it turned out, the health message that Butler had produced need not have been delivered, for the White House health work group recommended the selection of the third alternative presented in the memorandum to Ehrlichman. The work group also told Butler that even though it had been decided there would be no formal Presidential health message in 1970, the matter could not simply be dropped. HEW had to say something.

During that last frantic week before the health memorandum was sent over to the White House, both Butler and Veneman realized that events were fortuitously moving in their direction. Veneman was already on Capitol Hill testifying on various sections of the Administration's welfare reform proposal; and on Monday, March 23, the legislators were to go into executive session on Medicare and Medicaid. The President's options as drafted by Butler, working with Ellwood and the Minneapolis group, offered no presentations to the White House that did not include the health maintenance approach. The proposed choices were to have the President go with HMOs, or have the President endorse HEW going with HMOs, or have HEW go with HMOs alone. There were no other choices. Because the White House had to present a health initiative, Butler and Veneman artfully capitalized on the situation by seeing to it that the only initiative available was HMO. Not surprisingly, then, the White House gave HEW its blessings to go forward with the HMO (Part C) initiative on Capitol Hill and to publicize this initiative.

Part C Goes to Capitol Hill

While it was Butler's responsibility to cover the White House for HEW, it was Under Secretary Veneman's responsibility to relate to Capitol Hill. In fact, Veneman had been on Capitol Hill virtually every day since November presenting the Administration's Family Assistance Program (FAP) to the House Ways and Means Committee. The idea for a Part C HMO option for Medicare, then, was a logical extension of the total FAP proposal. Medicare and Medicaid, after all, were part of the same Social Security Act that institutionalized the federal/state welfare system. Medicaid, in particular, was nothing more than a health component of the federal/state welfare system.

As the HMO proposal began to develop under Butler's leadership, Veneman saw that the timing for the emergence of the proposal and the flow of events before the Ways and Means Committee on Capitol Hill were converging quite nicely. The availability of the Ways and Means Committee as an appropriate and convenient forum for launching the Administration's HMO initiative — without requiring a major Presidential endorsement — was indeed a fortuitous circumstance. Veneman, then, began to urge Butler to make something available for him to bring before the Ways and Means Committee in the waning days of the executive session on Social Security amendments.

On Monday, March 23, the last two days of the executive session of the Ways and Means Committee hearings on welfare reform began. Committee Chairman Wilbur Mills and his colleagues were in the process of reviewing the Medicare and Medicaid program. Prior to the March 23 session, Veneman had talked privately to Mills, to John Byrnes, the minority senior member, and to John Martin, the chief counsel of Ways and Means, indicating to them that this new idea called HMO, the Part C option, was available and that the Administration would like to present it. Toward the close of the Monday, March 23, session, Veneman brought the HMO Part C idea formally to the attention of the Committee and, toward the end of the following day's session, which was to be the last, Mills turned to Veneman and said, "OK, we've marked up the bill. Is there anything else? Veneman replied, "Well, Mr. Chairman, that discussion yesterday about Part C for Medicare — what's the general thought about that?" Mills said, "That's fine. Nobody's got any objection to that, do they?"[31] The last 15 minutes of three months of executive sessions on the entire welfare reform package was not a time for lengthy contemplation of new proposals. The committee was in a hurry to con-

31. John G. Veneman, interview, Nov. 1973. Veneman reconstructed the conversation as he remembered it.

clude, and Mills was, of course, marking up the bill. So, with no discussion at all, Mills routinely inserted the Part C proposal into the marked-up bill. Veneman then asked Mills if he would mind if HEW put out a public statement on the HMO Part C proposal. Mills had no objection. Veneman returned to his office that night and told Butler that it was all right to go ahead with a public statement.

HEW Announces the Health Maintenance Strategy

On Wednesday, March 25, HEW Secretary Finch issued a statement announcing the Part C HMO option. Simultaneously, an HEW press release left no doubt that the cornerstone of the new Administration policy was the health maintenance plan:

> The key to the announced long-range strategy is the increased use of annual health maintenance contracts. The Secretary announced that legislation would be proposed to authorize the Social Security Administration to enter into such contracts guaranteeing comprehensive health services for the elderly at a fixed annual rate. Our goal, the Secretary said, is that every elderly or poor person, covered by Medicare or Medicaid, be given the right to choose between receiving services under such a contract and receiving individual hospital and physician services in the traditional manner. We must promote diversity, choice, and healthy competition in American Medicine if we are to escape from the grip of spiralling costs.[32]

Under Secretary Veneman followed up the public announcement with a memorandum on the health maintenance option to a long list of directors of health-related offices in HEW. This memorandum highlighted key points in Finch's March 25 statement, made it clear that the cornerstone of the Administration's health policy was the health maintenance contract through the vehicles of Medicare and Medicaid payments, and made preliminary management assignments.[33] Now that the Administration had formally committed itself to the health maintenance strategy, it had to face the challenge of realizing its program. All that had been accomplished up to March 25, 1970, was at the level of policy and philosophy. The initiative now moved to the ongoing health bureaus of HEW and to the Congress.

---

32. Press release, Department of Health, Education, and Welfare, Mar. 25, 1970.
33. John G. Veneman, "The Health Maintenance Option," memorandum from the Under Secretary, HEW, Apr. 8, 1970.

CHAPTER 3

A Cornerstone of National Health Policy

The health maintenance plan was anything but a fully developed policy when it was presented to the White House over the persistent opposition of HEW's professional health bureaucrats. The White House announcement was a signal that the HMO initiative enjoyed only conditional approval. The plan's immediate fate would depend on how well HEW's top leadership sustained the momentum generated by health maintenance and whether reluctant health careerists would now join in and vigorously support the health maintenance plan as their own.

The Institutional Framework

On March 31, 1970, Under Secretary John Veneman established the Health Finance and Delivery Reform Project Group, under the leadership of James ("Jamie") McLane, a special assistant to Secretary Finch. The project group's purpose was "to redeploy present resources to stimulate and improve the organization and delivery of health services, with primary emphasis on HMOs."[1] The project group was staffed by the Management Planning Group, composed primarily of a bright, young cadre of management specialists (MBAs) recruited to HEW by Deputy

1. John G. Veneman, "Management of the Health Maintenance Project," memorandum to the Secretary, Department of Health, Education, and Welfare (DHEW)/Office of the Secretary (OS), Mar. 31, 1970.

Under Secretary Frederick Malek.[2] In the following months this cadre came to embrace health maintenance enthusiastically, and, in so doing, conflicted sharply with more cautious and circumspect members of the professional health bureaucracies. As broad objectives were tested for their programmatic potential, a fundamental issue emerged: was health maintenance to be an overarching — if not *the* overarching — health policy of the Nixon Administration, as the Management Planning Group perceived it? Or was it just another categorical program to be implemented co-equally with all of the others run by HEW?

The first step was to develop an implementation plan. McLane established a loosely knit task force composed of representatives from the agencies that would have chief responsibility for implementing an HMO program: the Health Services and Mental Health Administration (HSMHA), the Social Security Administration (SSA), and the Medical Services Administration (MSA). These individuals, in turn, headed up work groups in their own agencies. HSMHA, in particular, moved vigorously during this period under the guidance of Beverlee Myers, the assistant administrator for resource development. By early June, Myers and her staff had produced a large notebook full of background materials on such diverse topics as consumers and HMOs, monitoring HMOs, and HMO research.

Meanwhile, Paul Ellwood and his staff at the Minneapolis-based American Rehabilitation Foundation, struggled with a number of complex issues as they tried to spell out in greater detail the kinds of health care organizations that could be called HMOs. Because the matter was purposely vague in the original health maintenance plan, the range of organizations and services to be stimulated by the government would now have to be clearly identified.

Two essential tracks emerged: one was the composition of a legislative package; the other was an analysis of the actions the federal government could take, without benefit of further legislation, to implement the health maintenance plan. The difference between these two tracks very early highlighted a fundamental cleavage between the management analysts of Malek's Management Planning Group and the health planners and administrators in the Office of the Secretary and in the health bureaus. The Management Planning Group saw the HMO option as a vehicle for

---

2. Malek was to gain notoriety later as the Nixon Administration's personnel director and as a deputy director of the Office of Management and Budget. A graduate of the Harvard Business School, Malek was a prototype for the young business school graduates brought into government under the Republican administration.

government to stimulate the health care "marketplace" to behave in more efficient and productive ways. This would mean publicizing, prodding, and, ultimately, offering technical assistance to groups interested in establishing HMOs. Insurance companies, in particular, were likely candidates for this kind of activity, and profit-making HMOs would be actively encouraged.

As one of the Management Planning Group professionals put it:

> Everyone in the government is so concerned about getting a piece of legislation passed, they think that's the only way you change anything. . . . That's flat wrong. Everyone was so uptight to get a piece of legislation and testifying and writing the Secretary's testimony . . . that no one was concerned with the substance of making change happen in the health delivery system. . . . The Management Planning Group's view of the world . . . was more getting something done with existing resources by giving people responsibility. . . .

Much of this work could be accomplished without additional legislation. Thus, a principal objective of McLane, who also reflected this management perspective, was to lay out an aggressive work plan that would set up a variety of nonlegislative activities, oriented toward the private health sector.

Senior health planners in the Office of the Secretary and in HSMHA, however, had quite a different point of view. The former group was oriented toward the legislative process and the writing of health regulations, rather than toward the "technical assistance/facilitator" role reflected in the Management Planning Group's perspective. The latter group in HSMHA, although comfortable with a technical assistance role, was oriented primarily toward the not-for-profit, voluntary health care sector. This was, after all, where it did most of its business: giving out categorical grants-in-aid to university medical centers, voluntary and municipal hospitals, maternal and child health centers, and also to a few not-for-profit group practice plans. The idea of stimulating a competitive, private health care marketplace challenged HSMHA's traditional role.

SSA's early efforts, led by Bureau of Health Insurance (BHI) staff, was to begin to specify, in great detail, possible regulations to monitor the reimbursement of HMOs. The Part C proposal called for the reimbursement of hospitals and physicians on the basis of a prenegotiated price, requiring BHI to refocus its established "customary, usual, and reasonable" cost reimbursement practices. The term *prospective reim-*

bursement was proposed as a way of indicating that dollars might be advanced to HMOs, on the condition that retroactive adjustments would be made on the basis of cost experiences. The idea of a reimbursement mechanism based solely on price would not be accepted.

It was clear to Ellwood and other HMO advocates that BHI was taking an excessively restrictive stance on HMOs. Having lost the earlier battle to kill health maintenance in March, one view of BHI behavior had the bureau fighting a rearguard holding action. On balance, BHI's conservatism clashed sharply with the market incentive concept behind the health maintenance strategy.

By the spring of 1970, the principal governmental actors in the unfolding health maintenance drama had already begun to shape the emerging program in their own images. HSMHA focused on program specifications (what would HMOs look like); BHI focused on payment mechanism controls (how to ensure that the public trust would not be served badly by prepayment); and the Management Planning Group began to stimulate private sector interest in forming HMOs.[3]

Slow Beginnings

McLane provided the fledgling HMO implementation effort with strong leadership during these early months. He realized that unless the process were ultimately institutionalized in the bureaucracies, there would be continuing resistance. Thus, a major reason for establishing an interagency task force very early was to win over or neutralize potential centers of opposition to the common departmental purpose. However, a new policy initiative could be sustained through existing bureaucratic resources only if a firm commitment was elicited from the participants: HSMHA, BHI, and MSA. The momentum could be maintained as long as it was perceived that a high priority was being placed on the effort by HEW's top leadership.

McLane was able to sustain a reasonable level of commitment through the early summer months of 1970. The culmination of this effort was his "Work Plan for Implementing the Health Maintenance Option," presented to the Under Secretary and other HEW staff on July 31, 1970. The plan specified nine task areas, allocated assignments among the bureaus, and, in McLane's own words, "has been developed to ensure implemen-

---

3. The Medical Services Administration (MSA), which administered the Medicaid program, was also a key agency involved in early HMO policy deliberations. MSA was very supportive of the Health Maintenance Strategy, seeing an important opportunity to play the "high" policy game, as well as to improve Medicaid cost control.

tation of the HMO option by January 1, 1971."[4] Working on the assumption that "Part C would be through the Senate Finance Committee" in "another month or two," McLane declared that "We must move ahead on the positive assumption that this option or something like it will pass the Senate." His timetable, as it turned out, was exactly two years ahead of schedule. Not only did the work plan seriously overestimate the enthusiasm of the U.S. Senate for HMOs, it also overestimated both the capacity and the willingness of HEW's own health bureaus to sustain the effort.

The implementation plan never became fully operational. McLane left HEW in early August, and the HMO project then came under the leadership of Deputy Assistant Secretary for Health and Scientific Affairs James Cavanaugh. A number of simultaneous occurrences signaled the breakdown of the HMO implementation process during the late summer and fall of 1970.

A Call for National Health Policy

A Presidential health message had been planned for March 1970, but, at the last minute, it was deferred in favor of Finch's announcement of the HMO initiative. The White House began to show renewed interest in health almost immediately, as a direct result of the difficulties encountered by the Family Assistance Plan during Senate Finance Committee hearings in April. When chided for the large "notches" remaining in the welfare system because such programs as Medicaid were not folded into a uniform program, the Administration promised to revise its approach to financing health services for the poor.[5]

Then in early July, in response to a White House request to provide "a rough summary of some of the options open to us in developing a health strategy for 1971," Butler submitted a summary of "Health Options, 1971." After reviewing this paper, Edward Morgan, Presidential adviser John Ehrlichman's deputy on the White House staff, suggested to Butler that the next step might be for HEW to prepare, officially, its analysis of various alternative health strategies. "Morgan indicated that the President has a growing interest in health. . . ."[6]

4. James W. McLane, "Work Plan for Implementing Health Maintenance Organization Option," DHEW/OS, July 31, 1970.
5. "Notches" are illogical gaps in the structure of a uniform system of welfare payments caused by the categorical coverage of a particular benefit not folded into the uniform system of coverage. The effects of notches can be either to double cover a particular benefit or to allow a benefit to fall through the cracks of a uniform payment program.
6. Lewis Butler, "Health Strategy — White House Interest," memorandum to the Secretary, DHEW/OS, July 21, 1970.

In late July, Ehrlichman asked Secretary of Health, Education, and Welfare Elliot L. Richardson to "begin to prepare a comprehensive analysis of this issue."[7] Ehrlichman noted that "Attached is a preliminary index of possible health options developed by the Domestic Council staff in cooperation with your department." This index was the paper sent to Morgan by Butler, now being routed back to the Secretary via the White House.

Deputy Under Secretary Robert Patricelli indicated that Ehrlichman was not asking for "specific legislative proposals" at this time. Moreover, he said, the memo from Ehrlichman:

> . . . was sent as an "accident"; Morgan had prepared the draft as a model to ask Ehrlichman if that was how he wanted to deal with the Departments under the Domestic Council setup. It was to be discussed with Domestic Council staff, but was sent out by Ehrlichman.[8]

These exchanges comprise the ingredients for a comic opera. They show just how unwieldy was the machinery established to coordinate policy formulation through the new Domestic Council. The health policy process for fiscal year 1971 had commenced, if in a somewhat awkward manner.

A timetable and a work program for producing the President's health policy options were established in early August. Two components were set in motion: the Family Health Insurance Plan (FHIP) development process and the Health Options process. FHIP's broad outline had been announced by the President in early June as "the nation's first federally subsidized system of health insurance for the poor."[9] Paradoxically, then, the Nixon Administration's position that a national health insurance plan would be excessively inflationary had to be modified in order to conform extant welfare categories to the structure of the Administration's welfare reform program. The Medicaid program would have to be federalized for the sake of consistency. Later, FHIP could be broadened to cover the entire population.

---

7. John Ehrlichman, memorandum to Secretary Richardson, the White House, July 21, 1970.
8. Robert E. Patricelli, "Scenario on Development of FHIP and Health Policy Options," memorandum to the Secretary, DHEW/OS, Aug. 3, 1970.
9. John Osborne, quoted from the New Republic, in: Daniel P. Moynihan. *The Politics of a Guaranteed Income: The Nixon Administration and the Family Assistance Plan.* New York City: Random House, Inc., 1973.

In August, two large work groups were established: one for Finance Options, the other for Health Options. Assistant Secretary for Health and Scientific Affairs Roger O. Egeberg, M.D., was to coordinate the Health Options process, mobilizing the resources of HSMHA, the National Institutes of Health (NIH), the Food and Drug Administration (FDA), and the Environmental Health Service (EHS).

Health Maintenance Gets Lost in the Swamp

The Health Options process sidetracked the nascent HMO initiative. Walter McClure, a key member of Ellwood's Minneapolis-based staff, prophetically warned:

> I think we should be putting some thought to what should go into the Nixon address next year and how we should get it there. The dangers of not inputting are that he may come up with some proposals that are unrealistic or impractical or that do not meet the real problems, and that health maintenance may get lost in the swamp.[10]

Ellwood concurred a month later, observing that the Health Options process "is a fiasco. No one caught the signal. HMO is the name of the game."[11] Over the next two months, Ellwood and members of HEW's Health Finance and Delivery Reform Project Group staff struggled to keep HMO afloat amid a maze of bureaucratic options, drafts and redrafts, that emerged from the Health Options process.

The "swamp" foreseen by McClure was really created by circumstances inherent in the structure and style of decision making in HEW. Rather than an orderly system of policy making, HEW in 1970 presented little more than an amorphous clustering of ad hoc work groups, poorly organized agencies, personalities, styles, and, as one observer noted, free lancers. Whatever the intellectual brilliance of top HEW leadership, it had clearly sacrificed orderly process and agency morale for the more frenetic approach of ad hoc work groups, outside consultants, and overt encouragement of individual entrepreneurship. In just 18 months, HEW had developed two bold departures in social welfare and health policy (the Family Assistance Plan and HMO); but, paradoxically, the permanent agencies and bureaus found themselves left out and demoralized. Finch succumbed to this chaotic process and

---

10. Walter McClure, "Thoughts on Nixon's Health Policy Address," Institute for Interdisciplinary Studies, Aug. 26, 1970.
11. Paul M. Ellwood Jr., M.D., notes, Sept. 30, 1970.

abruptly resigned as HEW Secretary in June to become a counselor to the President.[12]

Elliot Richardson became HEW Secretary in June 1970, with a palace revolt on his hands at the agency level and overt jockeying for position and influence among his own senior staff. The Health Options process could serve a useful purpose by structuring some order out of this chaos. The Health Options effort could also tap the creative impulses in the bureaus (if creativity and bureaucracy could be harmonized).

Richardson officially launched the new process for health policy development early in August, establishing the Finance work group and the Health Options work group. His timetable called for about a one month's effort to pull the proposals from each group together. Work on the Finance Options proceeded smoothly, coordinated by Lewis Butler, assistant secretary for planning and evaluation, and Ruth Hanft, Butler's chief health aide, working with SSA. But on the Health Options side, no small inner core of analysts took responsibility.

Within a month, Egeberg could proudly report that over 60 people had been mobilized for the effort. In all, two volumes of options were produced, some 250 all told. After getting a look at these materials, a senior OMB official with top-level coordinating responsibilities concluded: ". . . the health options book was one of the worst pieces of work I have ever seen from a government agency. Pages in it were upside down; it was really terrible."[13]

OMB and White House officials, alarmed at this in-process work, began to make plans to establish yet another White House-level health work group — similar to the one established in 1969 — this time as a committee of the new Domestic Council.

Health Maintenance Emerges from the Swamp

The Health Options process was, by now, well beyond the original deadlines established in August 1970. It was mid-October and the Secretary's report to the President was only just being drawn out of a broad array of options. This extended time frame, however, gave the ad-

---

12. The theme of "creativity out of chaos" is, perhaps, endemic to any unwieldy bureaucratic system. In hindsight, Finch may not have managed HEW very well, but he sparked rapid innovations in social policy, largely by ignoring the bureaucracies, incurring their enmity along the way.
13. Without detailed guidance from the Secretary as to format and purpose, it was inevitable that the Health Options process would fall of its own weight. With so many actors involved, from the health agencies, there was no chance that a coherent policy analysis would have been conducted.

vocates of health maintenance the opportunity they needed to pull their concept out from among the 250 other options. Richardson proved a willing ally in this resurrection.

When Richardson came to HEW in June, one of his first acts as Secretary was to testify in support of the Medicare HMO option to H.R. 17550 before the Senate Finance Committee. He did not need to be convinced of the virtues of the HMO approach and was, from the beginning, an unwavering supporter of the policy. His concept of HMO was extremely ecumenical:

> I adhered from the outset to a definition of an HMO, namely that it is any arrangement which has the function of allocating prepaid dollars over the whole range, a comprehensive range of needed health services. The only thing that an HMO does for you is to create a point at which somebody has to look at how dollars are distributed.[14]

Even after becoming preoccupied with the broad Health Options process, Richardson showed continuing interest in health maintenance. Toward the end of September, he asked Deputy Assistant Secretary James Cavanaugh, nominally in charge of the ongoing HMO-oriented Health Finance and Delivery Reform Project Group, "whether or not we are doing enough within our existing resources to provide incentives for the development of Health Maintenance Organizations."[15] The question was opportune and reflected the growing concern of members of the miniscule HMO project group in Under Secretary Veneman's office that Cavanaugh was dragging his feet on HMOs. In fact, Veneman had been alerted by members of the Health Finance and Delivery Reform Project Group staff that the HMO effort was in trouble.

Meanwhile, Deputy Under Secretary Patricelli had the unenviable task of shaping the materials produced by the FHIP and Health Options task forces into a coherent series of health policy papers that the Secretary would present to the President. Given the poor quality of the Health Options materials, Patricelli was left to weave a silk purse out of a sow's ear. In late September, he requested that a list of "hot options" and an outline for decision papers for each option be developed. Egeberg's response arrived in mid-October. It was a 19-page outline and, on page 12, at the bottom, appeared "Health Maintenace Organizations" under the

---

14. Elliot L. Richardson, interview, July 1974.
15. James H. Cavanaugh, "Progress on Health Maintenance Organizations," memorandum from the Deputy Assistant Secretary for Health and Scientific Affairs to the Secretary, Oct. 9, 1970.

amorphous heading "Options To Encourage the Use of Lower-Cost Resources and Promote Economies of Scale." A short "HMO option" was attached as a tab to the outline.

Patricelli realized that much further work would have to be done if high-quality decision papers were to be produced. Therefore, he called on the Health Finance and Delivery Reform Project Group to produce a fully developed HMO option at almost the identical time that the Secretary made his pointed inquiry about progress on HMOs. A special work group was convened and this activity merged with Cavanaugh's efforts to rekindle action on HMOs in response to Richardson's query.

Early in October, Cavanaugh observed in a memo to HSMHA Administrator Vernon E. Wilson that "Secretary Richardson has not only reaffirmed his support of the HMO concept but has questioned whether HEW is doing enough to encourage the formation of HMOs." Cavanaugh charged HSMHA with "lead agency" responsibility for developing an information brochure for distribution to potential HMO organizers, developing an in-house capacity to provide technical assistance to groups interested in forming HMOs, development of a monitoring capacity to discriminate among HMOs in terms of their relative efficiency and effectiveness, development of an HMO research program, and, finally, input into regulations design.[16]

Cavanaugh's charge to Wilson reinforced Wilson's own desire and perception that HSMHA ought to be in charge of HEW's HMO effort. However, this apparent mandate was upsetting to the HMO project group in Veneman's office. They pointed out that "Jim, apparently inadvertently, has given Dr. Wilson the idea that he will be leading the HMO effort for the Department."[17] Veneman's staff advocated that strong and vigorous leadership be maintained in the Health Finance and Delivery Reform Project Group in the Office of the Secretary.

The problem lay in the ambiguity of the term *lead agency*. Did it mean taking the lead only in those areas assigned to HSMHA? Or, was the mandate from Cavanaugh meant to be broader? The charge could be read either way. Although Cavanaugh gave Wilson a specific scope of work to follow, it was certainly broad enough to be considered as encompassing the entire HMO development effort. Wilson chose to interpret his mandate broadly, placing it in direct conflict with the mandate given

16. James H. Cavanaugh, Untitled memorandum to Vernon E. Wilson, M.D., Administrator, HSMHA, DHEW/OS, Oct. 7, 1970.
17. Unsigned memorandum to the Under Secretary, Oct. 26, 1970.

the Health Finance and Delivery Reform Project Group by Veneman in March.

The enthusiasm of the health maintenance advocates in the Under Secretary's Office now came into direct conflict with the more cautious view of HSMHA. HSMHA presented a draft HMO option, which, for the first time, called for a serious developmental effort involving federal funds to capitalize HMO starts. In all, about 1,300 HMOs covering a population base of 65 million persons, each serving an enrollment of 50,000 persons, could be developed over five years for a total cost of $500 million.[18] The Health Finance and Delivery Reform Project Group staff, however, believed these estimates to be far too timid. They, therefore, set out to rework the HMO presentation and, in early December, proposed a combination of options, some of them representing HSMHA's thinking and others reflecting their own. HSMHA'S "1,300 HMOs to be developed over five years" proposal was scrapped in favor of a far more expansive projection of between 5,000 and 10,000 HMOs plus a proposal that "serious consideration be given to converting a good portion of the 7,000 acute care hospitals in the country into HMOs."[19]

HSMHA reacted negatively to the revised HMO option, believing it to be too ambitious and unrealistic. "Our view is that 5,000 to 10,000 HMOs is a very ambitious goal, requiring perhaps a decade or more to reach."[20]

A Decision To Push Forward

The next steps were up to Richardson. A full-scale review was held in the HEW Chart Room in mid-December. The Secretary again restated the high priority he placed on the department's HMO effort. He asked for a

---

18. HSMHA, HMO Option Paper, Dec. 1970.
19. James H. Cavanaugh, "HMO Health Option," memorandum from the Deputy Assistant Secretary for Health and Scientific Affairs to the Secretary, DHEW/OS, Dec. 4, 1970. The 7,000 U.S. hospitals include all types of care. About 3,000 of these are specialized institutions.
20. Vernon E. Wilson, M.D., "Health Option HMO Paper," memorandum from the HSMHA Administrator to the Deputy Assistant Secretary for Health and Scientific Affairs, Dec. 8, 1970. Neither HSMHA nor BHI seemed to understand, even at this rather late date, that the health maintenance strategy was intended to be a long-range, comprehensive national health policy. Thus, earlier criticisms by HEW senior health planners and BHI staff that health maintenance was an ambitious 10-20 year plan, as well as Wilson's similar argument in December, could be viewed as the strength of health maintenance, not its weakness.

    On the other hand, with the hindsight of intervening years, all of these projections turned out to be wildly optimistic, grossly underestimating the political barriers to establishing HMOs as a serious alternative to fee-for-service medicine.

review of things that could be done "now," without new legislation. Present authority for incentive reimbursements under Titles XVIII and XIX, the Hill-Burton Health Facilities Construction program, and HSMHA's available grant programs (specifically, PHS Act section 314(e), demonstration projects, and section 304, National Center for Health Services Research and Development authorizations) were all mentioned as possible mechanisms for HMO development support. These authorities plus use of a model state law to reduce legal barriers to HMO formation were mechanisms with sufficient flexibility to accommodate the new HMO initiative.

The remainder of the meeting was focused on the need for governmental front-end capital funds to stimulate a market for HMOs. Available data pointed to very high start-up costs, probably about $1 million per HMO, over the first three years.

While no resolution of issues was achieved at the meeting, the areas of focus for HEW were clearly specified. And Richardson told participants that they would proceed regardless of the outcome of the legislation before the Senate.

On December 15, 1970, the Secretary reinforced his aggressive stance with regard to HMO in a memorandum, which stated:

> The more I have been exposed to the HMO concept, the more impressed I am by the conclusion that this is an initiative to which we should give the highest priority.

Then Richardson pointedly gave his senior staff and the health bureaucracies unequivocal marching orders:

> The fortunes of the HMO legislation before the current session of Congress do not, of course, affect in any way this effort. I want to emphasize the importance of moving ahead now with the development of the HMO concept. The new organizational incentives which are introduced by HMOs are of such fundamental importance to a restructuring of the public and private health industry that I do not feel we can await passage to expand our developmental activities.[21]

These expanded development activities would include four areas: policy coordination, funding initiatives, external relations, and development activities. The Secretary called on his controller and general counsel to explore and to reprogram existing grant authorities for HMOs and to

---

21. Elliot L. Richardson, "Health Maintenance Organizations (HMOs)," memorandum from the Secretary, DHEW/OS, Dec. 15, 1970.

develop programs of loans, loan guarantees, and possibly trust funds in order to cover initial operating deficits. HSMHA, in turn, would establish a grants program to administer reprogrammed funds and would provide technical assistance to potential HMO developers.

A revitalized HMO Working Group was established in the Under Secretary's office with Samuel "Sandy" Hale in charge. The Under Secretary transmitted the Secretary's memorandum and called for the submission of time-phased game plans to Hale by "close of business December 21."

The President's Health Message

The Secretary's decision to push forward with a vigorous HMO development program on December 15 had a significant impact on the President's 1971 health initiatives. In particular, at the precise time that dialog with the White House was increasing, the Secretary had focused the attention of his senior aides on HMO. Deputy Under Secretary Patricelli, in particular, was given responsibility for HMO policy coordination, in addition to his ongoing responsibility to coordinate the Health Options process that was establishing the President's health policy agenda. Patricelli came to perceive the two policy development assignments as part of a conceptual whole. As the time for the actual drafting of the President's message approached, Patricelli focused on HMO as a cornerstone of the President's health policy.

Although Richardson's decision to move forward with HMO without explicit White House authorization was not without risk, in reality it was a risk worth taking because the White House itself had already signaled that it found much to favor in HMO. Beginning on November 18, the Domestic Council health working group had begun to draft its own comprehensive health policy position paper. The White House established the health working group as a subcommittee of the Domestic Council, in part to coordinate the flow of policy to the Oval Office and, in part, because there were serious questions in a number of minds about HEW's ability to produce the required policy. HEW's inability to organize its health policy generating machinery during the year just ending had not been forgotten. Richardson, on the other hand, was determined to exert control over the establishment of the Administration's health policy.

When the Domestic Council completed its paper on December 8, the document was sent to Richardson. Assistant Secretary Butler, acting as a liaison between HEW and the work group, saw to it that these White House policy options reflected HEW's evolving health financing and delivery system proposals. As Richard Nathan, the health working group chairman, noted:

> . . . [The paper] included an HMO proposal which was really all along something that everybody involved in the deliberations on health felt was a good idea. . . . Lew [Butler] made a good argument each time it came up. Lew could answer any questions well. Everyone felt that proposals should be made to provide seed money and clear away institutional barriers.[22]

Ehrlichman requested that the Secretary respond to a series of questions about the Domestic Council paper on December 14. Richardson, however, had other ideas. He was not about to respond to a health policy agenda established outside of his department by the Domestic Council, especially when most of the materials being used reflected staff work accomplished in HEW. Rather than responding to Ehrlichman's December 14 request, the Secretary sought an immediate meeting and, over lunch on December 15, Richardson told Ehrlichman that, in effect, the Vice-President, who nominally chaired the Domestic Council health policy review of which the health working group was a staff operation,

> . . . wanted to go back to square one on everything. And I said that we just couldn't get there. . . . There would be no health message . . . and Ehrlichman agreed with this. It was left that I would develop a memorandum for him to look at which would issue instructions to various people to get this done. I drafted a memorandum . . . and it came back [from Ehrlichman] exclusively to me, giving me full responsibility for the development of the package from that point forward. And it shunted the Vice-President out of the picture.[23]

The following day, on December 16, Richardson submitted draft language to Ehrlichman, and on December 23 he had his mandate to prepare the President's health message. Ehrlichman told the Secretary, "The responsibility for the preparation and interagency coordination of all related papers, including the Brandeis Brief and the first draft of the President's message to Congress, is yours."[24]

From that point forward, it was a virtual certainty that health maintenance would be the high point of the President's health message. Richardson had already committed HEW to a major HMO developmen-

---

22. Richard Nathan, interview, Mar. 1974.
23. Elliot L. Richardson, interview, July 1974.
24. John Ehrlichman, memorandum to Secretary Richardson, the White House, Dec. 23, 1970.

tal effort; now, he would substantially control the agenda for the President's health message.

On December 31, the Secretary sent to the President, ". . . a decision paper posing what I think are the key health policy issues which you need to decide to guide our future work."[25] Decision Issue 7 was "Support for Health Maintenance Organizations." Richardson reminded the White House, somewhat obliquely, that he, not Domestic Council and OMB staff, was in charge of the effort:

> Pursuant to John Ehrlichman's memorandum of December 23, I was given responsibility for preparing this memorandum. We have had the valuable assistance of Domestic Council and OMB staff in this effort, but the responsibility for the product is the Department's.

The President's response to Richardson's health decision paper arrived on January 5, 1971. There were a number of surprises, disclosing that HMO was not yet firmly in place on the President's health policy agenda:

> The proposal to encourage the formation of Health Maintenance Organizations, particularly in medically underserved areas, through a four-year program including federal loan guarantees, direct loans, project grants, and preferential reimbursement rates under government insurance will remain an open question subject to further work with OMB on reprogramming and grant consolidation possibilities. It is possible that we will want to experiment with a few before embarking on a full program.[26]

Then came this request: "The President has requested that a proposal be prepared outlining options for developing up to 800 neighborhood health centers (NHCs) in the next three to six years."

Using his direct access to the President, Donald Rumsfeld, a counselor to the President and formerly the director of the Office of Economic Opportunity (OEO), had slipped a counterproposal past Secretary Richardson and gained access to the emerging health policy agenda. Rumsfeld was concerned about the access of the poor to health services. HMOs were not designed to help the poor; they were essentially programs for the middle class. Without an expanded complement of NHCs to take advantage of the prepayment opportunities afforded by

---

25. Elliot L. Richardson, memorandum for the President, DHEW/Office of the Secretary, Dec. 31, 1970.
26. John Ehrlichman, memorandum to Secretary Richardson, the White House, Jan. 5, 1970.

the Family Health Insurance Plan, Rumsfeld reasoned that the Administration's health insurance proposal would have virtually ignored the poor.[27]

Whatever the merits of the Rumsfeld proposal, coming as it did at the 11th hour, it could only be viewed as yet another test of Richardson's ability to control the formulation of national health policy. The Secretary's senior staff set about to defend their hard-won prerogatives and the content of their emerging health policy.

The issue was not merely political, however. Fundamentally, the health maintenance approach was the antithesis of the categorical, piecemeal approach represented by the various NHC programs that had developed since 1965. HMOs were generic health delivery systems of many different types, one of which could be neighborhood health centers. The HMO approach was sufficiently comprehensive to encompass an NHC model, but NHCs were too narrowly conceived to accommodate varieties of HMOs. Thus, HEW could try to incorporate NHCs into its HMO proposal and, by so doing, co-opt OEO's opposition. This is the course of action HEW chose to follow.

OEO submitted a fully developed proposal calling for the establishment of over 800 "family health centers."[28] John Valiante, a management analyst in the Under Secretary's office, noted that there were three options for HEW to take with regard to the family health center (FHC) proposal.[29] OEO's preference would be to establish a separate corporation to build nearly 1,000 FHCs as a "brick and mortar" memorial to President Richard M. Nixon's concern for the health needs of the poor. A second option might be to build FHCs "under the umbrella of our HMO strategy in such a way that enables FHCs to become self-

---

27. In an entirely different context, the issue of appropriate health services availability was of primary concern to Sen. Edward Kennedy, when he took up the HMO question, in mid-1971. If HMOs were to be the delivery system complement to a national health insurance program, then it was essential that mandated HMO services be at least as comprehensive as those to be paid for by an insurance program. For Sen. Kennedy, this meant health service benefits identical to those to be covered by his Health Security Program. It would become readily apparent during the congressional debates that many people, including Donald Rumsfeld, saw HMO as an element of the larger national health insurance issue. They were not particularly concerned with the short-term issue of whether HMOs could compete in the present (admittedly) flawed marketplace, for NHI would solve the competitive problem legislatively.
28. *Family health centers* was the new term coined by the Nixon Administration to distinguish their neighborhood health centers from those of the earlier Democratic administration.
29. John Valiante, a member of the Health Finance and Delivery Reform Project Group in the Under Secretary's office, was doing much of the staff work on HMOs by the late fall of 1970.

sustaining from the start." A third option would be not to build FHCs at all, "on the basis that Neighborhood Health Centers have not clearly demonstrated their effectiveness."[30]

Valiante's discussion of the pros and cons of each of the three options leaves little doubt that he categorically opposed a distinctive FHC initiative and was somewhat less dubious, though dubious still, about an FHC option within HMO. As to the political arguments that FHCs were a fitting memorial in brick and mortar for Nixon, one of the Under Secretary's consultant's on HMO observed:

> A further claimed advantage of an accelerated NHC program is that: "The Democrats haven't preempted this area. There is no easy way they could 'one-up' us." I would have thought the very opposite. NHCs are, at least arguably, unadulterated Great Society, conceived and begun at the height of President Johnson's popularity. Rather than a Nixon initiative, the NHC effort could be construed as a return to the post-war Johnson-Kennedy interest in community programs. In any event, the President will have to explain why he terminated the burgeoning NHC program when he first took office.
>
> The final alleged advantage of NHCs — "tangible" or "hard" programs are good politically — also seems debatable. Clearly Johnson's "hard," "tangible" Vietnam policies . . . did not help our former President politically. It, therefore, seems to me that "hard" programs are not *a priori* good politics; it depends on the "hard" programs.[31]

On January 18, 1971, Richardson submitted to the President a decision paper including a distinct FHC option, a distinct HMO option, and an option folding FHCs into the broader HMO proposal. It was slightly revised and resubmitted on February 2.[32] First, the original HMO option was restated. It called for a developmental effort to establish 1,500 HMOs over a five-year period, offering enrollment to 40 million persons, and covering 90 percent of the population.[33] The program consisted of four parts: (1) a $250 million program of grants and contracts, which

---

30. John Valiante, "Family Health Centers," memorandum to the Deputy Under Secretary, Jan. 16, 1971.
31. Bruce Caputo, "Community Health Centers," memorandum to the Deputy Under Secretary, Jan. 7, 1971.
32. Elliot L. Richardson, memorandum for the President, Subject: Further Decision Issues on Health, DHEW/Office of the Secretary, Jan. 18, 1971, revised Feb. 2, 1971.
33. The earlier suggestion of the Health Finance and Delivery Reform Project Group for 5-10,000 HMOs had, by this time, been effectively temporized by the twin pressures of HSMHA's caution and the White House's unwillingness to commit vast sums of

could be made to any public, private, nonprofit, or profit-making organizations; (2) a loan guarantee program to underwrite loans secured from private sources to cover the costs of capital investments and initial operating deficits; (3) direct loans to public HMOs such as municipal or county hospitals or corporations that are not eligible for loan guarantees; and (4) operating grants to HMOs in areas of scarcity. Two additional elements, (1) special grants and contracts for transportation and outreach for poverty populations and (2) special grants to medical schools, were subsequently dropped.

The second option presented OEO's FHC proposal. Six arguments in favor of the proposal were discussed in a short and perfunctory manner. Nine elaborately reasoned negative arguments were presented, however. With HEW presenting both pro and con arguments, the Secretary could, in effect, weaken the FHC option by the very manner of his presentation. By controlling the agenda-setting mechanism for health policy, Richardson was able to marshal the strongest possible case against the OEO proposal.

Finally, a third option was offered, "A Combined Health Maintenance Organization and Family Health Center Strategy." Richardson recommended this approach:

> The Secretary recommends option 3 as a joint Health Maintenance Organization-Family Health Center strategy, supported by the new legislation called for.
>
> Whatever may be the decision on this issue, the Secretary strongly opposes the creation of a new Federal Corporation to manage a separate Family Health Center effort.
>
> This position is taken because:
>
> (1) Much of the financial support for FHCs would continue to come from HEW, raising extremely difficult problems of coordination of funding and regulatory policy.
>
> (2) . . . FHCs should be seen as part of a comprehensive strategy to create prepaid group practice institutions, together with HMOs. One piece of that strategy cannot effectively be administered apart from the rest.[34]

---

money to an HMO effort. In the Administration's white paper, entitled "Toward A Comprehensive Health Policy for the 1970s," U.S. Department of Health, Education, and Welfare, May 1971, p. 37, the final projection arrived at was 1,700 HMOs by fiscal year 1976.

34. Elliot L. Richardson, memorandum for the President, Subject: Further Decision Issues on Health, DHEW, Office of the Secretary, Jan. 18, 1971, revised Feb. 2, 1971.

The White House accepted Richardson's recommendation and HMO remained the central health delivery reform concept.

The final round of meetings and decision papers had all but concluded by the first week in February. The HMO proposal was firmly in place. All that remained were details and fine tuning. One such detail that would become a focus of controversy two years later was the Secretary's decision to commit the Administration to the preemption of legal barriers to HMOs through the exercise of federal supremacy in Medicare contracts and through the development of a model state law, which states could adopt, to eliminate legal barriers. The President accepted this recommendation.

The Vice-President, however, would have the next-to-last word. As the various decision options and Secretarial recommendations came out of HEW, they went back to the Domestic Council's health policy review group, chaired by Vice-President Spiro Agnew. Agnew had earlier expressed objections to the direction in which Richardson was taking national health policy. The Secretary, however, had received assurances at the time from Ehrlichman that he, Richardson, was in charge of the health policy development process.[35]

On February 11, 1971 the final Domestic Council briefing was held for the President in his office. Present were Nixon; Richardson; Kenneth Cole, deputy assistant to the President; George Shultz, the director of OMB; Richard Nathan; and Lewis Butler. The focus of the meeting was to get final Presidential decisions on the package of initiatives that would be the core of a Presidential health message and legislative proposals that would be recommended to the Congress.[36]

During the meeting, Cole was called away to take an urgent call from Agnew, then in California. Agnew again expressed his displeasure with the HMO proposal and asked Cole to put him through directly to the President. Cole agreed, and the President came on the line. "The Vice-President [told] the President that he was being misled by [Cole] and the

---

35. See pp. 57-59, this chapter, for a discussion of Richardson's insistence on full policy control in the matter of HMOs and overall health policy coordination.

36. During the fall, the original Family Health Insurance Plan (FHIP) had been expanded to cover the nonpoor under a National Health Insurance Standards Act (NHISA). Congressional interest in NHI had so quickened that the Administration felt compelled to develop its own program, calling for mandatory employee coverage, as part of employer fringe benefits. Both employer and employee would contribute to the premium and the program would be run through the private insurance carriers. NHISA was a "middle of the road" response to the more radical Kennedy Health Security Program.

others as to 'this HMO business' and it really didn't work and was a very bad deal for the President."[37]

Nixon responded that he would "talk to Ken about it." Cole prepared a briefing memo for the Vice-President, explaining why the HMO commitment did not mean that "the Federal Government would . . . be accepting an unlimited and very large financial commitment by endorsing an option to utilize HMOs. . . ."[38]

> I spent the better part of the weekend explaining to the Vice-President how [HMOs] weren't really that bad after all, and the plan had been recommended to the President, which the President had basically accepted. It was only a demonstration plan.
>
> . . . ultimately the President said go ahead with it, notwithstanding the Vice-President's objections, which was the President's job since he's the man who makes the decisions, not the Vice-President.[39]

The final obstacle to the HMO option had been overcome. Only the actual drafting of the Presidential message remained. That assignment fell to Patricelli and Lee Huebner, a Presidential speech writer. They were old friends from law school days at Harvard and the Ripon Society. Patricelli's initial draft and Huebner's own cut, however, reflected the lingering effects of the FHC initiative on the White House staff. Patricelli's version called for a health maintenance strategy as the organizing framework for the message. Heubner's version, which arrived at HEW on February 12, had substituted the phrase *family health center* for *health maintenance organization.* The description that followed was language defining HMOs, now summarily renamed FHCs by the White House. The HEW reaction was predictable and strong. Patricelli told Huebner that:

> Secretary Richardson feels very strongly that it would be a mistake to try to rename HMOs at this point. First, the name was coined by this Administration and has been widely accepted around the country. Second, it passed both House and Senate last year under this name and is now in H.R. 1. Third, HMOs are not "centers" or specific facilities, they are organizations; the FHC term is misleading on a basic point. Nor are HMOs limited to families. FHCs, as a name,

---

37. Kenneth R. Cole Jr., interview, Oct. 1974.
38. Kenneth R. Cole Jr., "HMOs," memorandum for the Vice-President, The White House, Feb. 13, 1971.
39. Kenneth R. Cole Jr., interview, Oct. 1974.

> should be retained for the new version of Neighborhood Health Centers; we don't want to have to go back to the poverty program title for them.[40]

HEW had its way. The President presented his health message to the Congress on February 18, 1971. The health maintenance strategy was its principal organizing theme and HMO was its principal organizational innovation.

The President began by reviewing the major problems in the health system. The chief problem was cost, but it was derivative from major health system failings, which had to be attacked comprehensively through a new "national health strategy," consisting of a six-point program. The first point in the program was reorganizing the delivery of service by increasing the availability of HMOs.

The President recalled that he had proposed "legislation last March to enable Medicare recipients to join such programs." He now called for four actions:

> 1. We should require public and private health insurance plans to allow beneficiaries to use their plan to purchase membership in a Health Maintenance Organization when one is available. . . .
> 2. To help new HMOs get started — an expensive and complicated task — we should establish a new $23 million program of planning grants to aid potential sponsors — in both the private and public sector.
> 3. At the same time, we should provide additional support to help sponsors raise the necessary capital . . . to sustain initial operating deficits until they achieve an enrollment which allows them to pay their own way. For this purpose, I propose a program of Federal loan guarantees, which will enable private sponsors to raise some $300 million in private loans during the first year of the program.
> 4. Other barriers to the development of HMOs include archaic laws in 22 States which prohibit or limit HMO development. I am instructing the Secretary of Health, Education, and Welfare to develop a model statute which the States themselves can adopt to correct these anomalies. In addition, the Federal Government will facilitate the development of HMOs in all States by entering into contracts with them to provide service to Medicare recipients and other Federal beneficiaries who elect such programs. Under

40. Robert Patricelli, "HEW Comments on Draft Health Message," DHEW/Office of the Secretary, Feb. 15, 1971.

> the supremacy clause to the Constitution these contracts will operate to preempt any inconsistent State statutes.[41]

The prominence of the health maintenance strategy and HMOs in the Presidential message was a singular event, given the obscurity of prepaid health care during the previous 40 years. Health maintenance arrived intact in the President's health message for three essential reasons.

First and foremost, HMO was an idea whose time had come; in fact, it was long past due. It was both comprehensive and compatible with the fundamental public-private nature of the extant health care system.

Second, the HMO concept was a politically attractive idea. It was untainted by previous Democratic initiatives and ideologically compatible with a posture of indirect rather than direct intervention into private marketplaces. Health maintenance, in short, was a conservative social reform, consistent with the "income approach" already devised for welfare reform. Unlike a "health centers approach," health maintenance could be presented as a phased withdrawal of direct federal intervention in the health care system, once initial capitalizing investments had been made.

Third, health maintenance generated an early and sustained advocacy and analytical capability, both within and outside of the Department of Health, Education, and Welfare. It had continuous and sustained support in the highest health policy circles. HEW leadership had been aided by Paul Ellwood and his staff at the American Rehabilitation Foundation, who moved about among the HEW bureaus and White House staff, providing educational and technical advice throughout the policy development process.

If there were any lingering doubts in the minds of the health bureaucrats of the Administration's seriousness about health maintenance, the Secretary's decision on December 15, 1970, to go forward before either legislative or full Presidential commitments had been secured ended their uncertainty. The President's message, in essence, was anticlimactic. The program could now go forward in earnest.

---

41. Richard M. Nixon, "National Health Strategy," the White House, Feb. 18, 1971.

CHAPTER 4

Implementation without Authorization

Secretary of Health, Education, and Welfare Elliot L. Richardson's decision on December 15, 1970, to move forward with the HMO development program anticipated the White House's full commitment to HMOs by two months. It also anticipated congressional commitment to HMOs by exactly three years. During that period of time, the Administration would utilize existing authorities in the Public Health and Social Security Acts to promote HMO development. Seventy-nine organizations would receive $16.5 million in grant funds before Congress officially authorized an HMO development program.[1] Richardson steadfastly maintained throughout this period that he had all the authority he needed to develop HMOs under existing law. Congress would eventually take a different point of view.

As the development program proceeded, the circle of interests perceiving the course of Administration policy as well as congressional activity would also widen. For, until the President put his full prestige behind HMOs, only a small circle of HEW officials, bureaucrats, and consultants were aware of the extent of the federal commitment. Now health interest groups, in particular the American Medical Association and the

1. George B. Strumpf and Marie A. Garramone. Why some HMOs develop slowly. *Public Health Reports*. 91:496, Nov.-Dec. 1976.

Group Health Association of America, began to measure the new policy against their own interests.[2]

Political interests and values take shape when policies become specific. At the level of generalities that had enveloped the early HMO debate within elite Administration circles, sufficient ambiguity existed to comfort a wide array of interests. For those who truly believed the rhetoric of market reform, HMOs would become a new competitive private-sector, profit-making component of the health services industry. Those who found such rhetoric somewhat dubious, however, took comfort in the fact that, after all, the Administration's entrepreneurial ardor would be constrained by the developmental tools at its disposal, that is, the existing grant-in-aid mechanisms that decidedly favored the not-for-profit sector.[3] And fiscal conservatives in the Social Security Administration could take heart in the fact that they would be controlling the pace of development of incentive reimbursement demonstrations under existing Social Security Act regulations.[4]

These institutional constraints notwithstanding, the Secretary gave his staff full authority to move forward. On January 6, 1971, a new HMO game plan was unveiled.

The New HMO Game Plan

The term *game plan* was much in vogue in the early years of the Nixon Administration, no doubt reflecting the Republican preoccupation with strategy, technique, and businesslike efficiency. The new HMO game plan identified the areas of activity to be undertaken during the remainder of fiscal year 1971, January through June. The Assistant Secretary/Controller would identify current funding sources and how to go about organizing them into an HMO development pool. Con-

---

2. See chapter 6, pp. 137-150, for an examination of AMA and GHAA strategies toward the emerging HMO policy.
3. "Grants" and "contracts" are the two most common instruments of federal health (fiscal) policy. Grants are awards only to public and private not-for-profit corporate entities. Contracts are often awarded to for-profit corporate entities, but usually for specific research and consultative activities. The stimulation of health services delivery is almost always through grants or, less frequently, through contracts to nonprofit and public organizations. If there is an interest in supporting health services development through profit-making entities, Congress restricts support to federal loans or loan guarantees.
4. The Part C HMO option would not pass into law until December 1972 when it emerged as Section 226 of the Social Security Amendments of 1972, Public Law 92-603. Until then, Section 402 of the Social Security Amendments of 1967, would guide prospective reimbursement demonstrations. The limited nature of this provision tended to reinforce SSA's cautious approach to promotion of prepayment.

gressional liaison would be carried forward on a continuing basis, in order to provide briefing materials for legislation then being drafted.[5] A major effort would be undertaken to publicize the Administration's HMO initiative through press briefings and meetings with national health, consumer, and labor organizations. Corporate investors who might be interested in starting HMOs with their own resources were to be contacted. An aggressive program to overcome state legal barriers to HMO formation would be undertaken, including the development of a model state law and a policy of withholding funds in "antigroup practice" states. A clearinghouse would be established to screen potential organizations for developmental funding. A program involving contracts with organizations that could undertake technical assistance and training activities would commence. Research projects to expand knowledge about HMOs would be undertaken by the National Center for Health Services Research and Development. And SSA would identify and undertake projects for incentive reimbursement demonstrations.

The Health Services and Mental Health Administration (HSMHA) reconstituted the HMO project group that had been working out of the planning and evaluation office in the office of the assistant administrator for resource development. A number of outside consultants were identified and, by March 1971, efforts were under way to bring them to HSMHA. A source of frustration to HSMHA Administrator Vernon Wilson and his senior staff was the reluctance of the Civil Service Commission to allow significant numbers of new staff positions to be created for an administrative unit without specific categorical legislative authority. Temporary "details" from other branches of the agency and temporary positions for outsiders were the short-term solutions to this problem.

Incentive Reimbursements and the Social Security Administration's Bureau of Health Insurance

The Bureau of Health Insurance (BHI) was, at best, a reluctant partner in the revitalized HMO game plan. At issue was the matter of how much latitude for experimentation was provided by the demonstration authority embodied in Section 402 of the Social Security Amendments of 1967. Deputy Commissioner Arthur E. Hess complained:

> There continues to be an optimism or an expectation that we can come forward with some magic interpretation of the incentive reim-

5. See chapters 5 and 6 for a full discussion of "The Legislative Struggle."

> bursement experiment authority. . . . This authority is, at best, extremely hedged about. . . .[6]

John Valiante, who now managed the HMO project office for the Under Secretary, was not satisfied with SSA's narrow interpretation of the statute. Therefore, he asked the HEW General Counsel to render an opinion on the scope of SSA's authority. Valiante also went out and asked officials of five HMOs if they would be interested in undertaking prepaid health care responsibility for Medicare enrollees. The response was positive.

The General Counsel concluded that SSA/BHI had the authority to engage in incentive reimbursement demonstrations without further legislation. Valiante proceeded to call a meeting with Hess, also attended by a member of the General Counsel's staff, who reinforced this affirmative ruling. SSA then began to move forward with the incentive reimbursement program, following up discussions with the five prepaid health plans indicating initial interest. The Office of General Counsel's ruling, however, complicated those discussions, since in its May 28 opinion it had also stated that only hospital-affiliated HMOs or HMOs owning hospitals could enter into incentive reimbursement agreements. Those HMOs that contracted out for their hospital services were ruled ineligible.

Meanwhile, a significant reformulation of the incentive reimbursement authority was being undertaken by the Senate Finance Committee. Coupled with the difficulties inherent in the General Counsel's ruling, the Finance Committee's deliberations provided BHI with all the evidence needed to table further work on HMO/Medicare contracts. BHI decided to await the outcome of pending legislation in the Congress, thereby effectively undermining HEW's attempts to utilize extant authority under the Social Security Act for HMO experimentation. The prospect of substantial enrollments of the elderly in HMOs would be delayed at least two years. Even after Public Law 92-603, the Social Security Amendments of 1972, became law in December 1972, an extended regulations-writing period delayed the process even longer.

One observer summarized the plight of HMO at the hands of the Social Security Administration:

> We are hard pressed to show that we got anything out of BHI this whole time. We got no money, no technical assistance, no incentive

---

6. Arthur E. Hess, memorandum regarding a forthcoming HMO Coordinating Committee meeting, SSA, Jan. 1971.

> reimbursements, experiments . . . nothing . . . but they sent a lot of people to meetings.

The real burden of HMO developmental efforts during this period was carried by HSMHA. HMO experienced a shaky beginning even there, however, as it struggled for resources and support among a large number of prior commitments and preemptive program priorities.

The HMO Development Program: First Grant Round

On February 19, 1971, Under Secretary John G. Veneman authorized a $6 million pooling of funds to support an HMO grant program. Five million dollars would come out of existing HSMHA authorizations, while $1 million would be provided through the Medicaid program.[7] Veneman's charge to HSMHA to reprogram these dollars for HMO development precipitated a great deal of activity within the agency. Which operating budgets would be tapped? How would decisions regarding the funding of projects be made?

The Under Secretary had accepted HSMHA's initial recommendations to tap $2.5 million from Section 304 (of the Public Health Service Act) funds administered by the National Center for Health Services Research and Development for the Experimental Health Services Delivery Systems (EHSDS) program.[8] Earlier, the Assistant General Counsel had ruled that Section 910(c) of Title IX of the PHS Act — establishing the Regional Medical Program (RMP) — would be available for HMO developmental efforts.[9] The only problem with using these funds during the remainder of fiscal year 1971 was that the Administration had impounded a substantial portion of RMP funds. To use this money now for HMO support would mean seeking OMB approval for its release.[10] That approval was not easily forthcoming, however, and Gerald Riso,

---

7. Section 1110 of the Social Security Act provides very broad authority for grants to states, public and for-profit organizations to support research or demonstration projects that will improve the effectiveness of programs "carried on or assisted under the Social Security Act and programs related thereto," and also provides for contracts with both nonprofit and profit-making organizations for these purposes.
8. The EHSDS was a demonstration effort to enable medical centers, comprehensive health planning agencies, and other medical care and health organizations to establish and evaluate new models in health care organization. Certainly, HMO demonstrations would qualify for funding under the EHSDS program.
9. Sidney Edelman, "HMO-Availability of Title IX Funds," memorandum to the HSMHA Administrator, HEW/OS/Office of the General Counsel, Dec. 21, 1970.
10. John G. Veneman, "Status Report on HMOs — Information Memorandum," memorandum from the Under Secretary to the Secretary, HEW/OS, Mar. 3, 1971.

a deputy assistant secretary for health and scientific affairs, clarified the request on March 19:

> If [the 2.5 million] are from RMP, this would be in accordance with the existing FY '71 obligational plan and would not involve the release of funds from reserve.[11]

Riso's clarification implied that the Secretary was then unwilling to make a case for the funds with OMB. He left no doubt that the additional $2.5 million would also have to come out of already obligated funds. The entire $5 million for HMO development would now have to be, as one observer noted, "torn out of HSMHA's hide to implement this program."

Reluctantly, Wilson turned away from RMP and decided to use obligations under Section 314(e) for community health services programs to fill out the $5 million HMO pool.

Wilson's efforts to identify the sources of the $5 million for HMO development and to establish a grant mechanism for the effort must be examined against three constraints. First and foremost was the difficulty in tapping resources already committed to other programs, despite the high priority placed on HMOs by the Secretary. Second was the administrative constraint, a priority of the HSMHA Administrator, to decentralize administrative procedures to regional offices, states, and localities. Because HMO was a new program, Wilson preferred a decentralized approach to program management involving a broad array of HSMHA program directors.

But the resource "tap," coupled with a decentralized administrative approach, led to a third, contradictory constraint: conflict with the time-phased milestones and aggressive stance taken by the HMO Project Office in the Secretary's office. Valiante, backed by Riso, who also served as vice-chairman of the HMO interdepartmental coordinating committee, exerted great pressure on Wilson. And, indeed, by the end of March, Wilson appeared to have gotten the HSMHA act together. An independent HMO staff office had been established, although the detailing of personnel from other programs was a frustrating process. Outside consultants were being brought in. And, finally, the elusive $5 million was found.

---

11. Gerald Riso, "HMO Funding," memorandum from Vice-Chairman, HMO Work Group to HSMHA Administrator, HEW/OS, Mar. 19, 1971. The term *reserve* was a polite reference to "impounded funds."

The tempo of activities increased during April. Wilson moved quickly to ready a grant round to be concluded by June. He notified his regional directors of the availability of the $1.2 million programmed to the regions and established procedures for the identification of potential applicants. In early June, the first grants and contracts for HMO development were awarded. Sixty-four projects were funded: 43 sponsored by 314(e), 6 by 304 (EHSDS) money, and 15 by Medicaid 1110 funds.[12] Clearly, the grant round had been organized in record time by Public Health Service bureaucratic standards.

Predictably, the HMO Project Office clashed sharply with its HSMHA counterparts over the appropriate focus of the grant program. Valiante typified the "downtown" point of view. As a newcomer to the health services field, he had not yet developed any strong opinions as to which kinds of HMO organizations might work better and, therefore, ought to be fostered by the federal government. His commitment was primarily to process, to getting a national demonstration program running as quickly as possible with a very broad array of organizations under federal sponsorship.[13]

The HSMHA-HMO leadership, however, emerged from contrasting professional training and experiences and, therefore, had developed different health service viewpoints. Beverlee Myers, the HSMHA-HMO acting director, and a Public Health Service career professional, had a definite preference for nonprofit prepaid group practice plans.[14] Valiante subsequently observed that, "Bev and I kept getting bogged down. . . . Her view of the model HMO was a consumer-sponsored Kaiser-like, nonprofit HMO run by an ex-Public Health Service type."

---

12. Howard Newman, the MSA commissioner, was eager to participate in the HMO development program. His contribution of $1 million to the effort was more symbolic of this commitment than significant. The grantees of the $1 million were really evaluation projects that bore only a passing resemblance to HMOs. In reality, then, only 49 projects were funded that had any possibility of reaching operational status. Newman's real contribution was to encourage states to negotiate prepayment contracts with Medicaid providers. In this, he was somewhat successful.
13. John Valiante's professional training was in business administration. He had been recruited to HEW's Management Planning Group by Deputy Under Secretary Frederick Malek, and reflected Malek's business management background and orientation. Gerald Riso, also recruited by Malek, had a similar perspective.
14. Beverlee Myers's training was in medical care administration. During the 1960s, Myers served in the Public Health Service and was closely associated with the Office of Group Practice Development, which was sponsoring small demonstrations with extant HMOs. The emphasis was entirely on prepaid group practice plans.

Myers, for her part, had a similar view of the pressures being exerted on her and HSMHA by Valiante and the HMO Project Office:

> Here was something which I personally had been pushing for years — prepaid group practice. And all of a sudden, it comes to the forefront and I'm very interested in it and I'm probably one of the more knowledgeable ones in the Public Health Service about it and I really thought it was great. Except, you know . . . the marketing aspect of it and some of the proprietary approaches, the profit-making organizations getting involved in it, went against my basic value judgments. . . . That is where some of the conflicts came at the staff level. . . . I never really had any problem with the basic concept of what it was we were trying to do. It was timing as well as some of the specific approaches. . . .[15]

Gordon MacLeod, M.D., who would shortly be tapped to direct the HSMHA effort, summarized the first grant round as follows:

> The first cycle was influenced strongly by the fact that they wanted to get something moving before the end of the fiscal year. And they called upon experienced hands to do this and . . . I thought they did an extraordinary job of getting a cycle in process. . . . It probably represented more the traditional bureaucracy approach to . . . traditional grant recipients [who] were prominent in the area, people who knew how to take grants out of the government.[16]

Riso, who was to play an important role in subsequent grant rounds, was less complimentary in his postmortem of the first grant round. He concluded it had severe limitations in demonstrating a broad range of strategic objectives. Throughout the spring of 1971, Valiante had complained that HSMHA was not moving quickly enough. Almost weekly, Riso would chair meetings among Veneman, Wilson, himself, and Valiante where the two protagonists — Valiante and Wilson — would clash over the course of program implementation. Valiante would express displeasure over HSMHA's apparent sluggishness, while Wilson would steadfastly maintain that the grant program was moving forward with deliberate speed.

The organizational ambiguity of the division of authority between the HMO Project Office and HSMHA clouded the substantive merits of the conflict. Riso came to see that there was more to it than a bitter personality conflict between the management specialist, Valiante, and the

---

15. Beverlee Myers, interview, July 1974.
16. Gordon MacLeod, M.D., interview, June 1974, p. 16.

senior physician administrator, Wilson. Valiante and Wilson actually reflected stark contrasts in organizational perspectives and institutional roles. Wilson viewed HMO from his position as HSMHA administrator: the program would move forward within the constraints of HSMHA's categorical programs. Valiante, on the other hand, viewed these constraints as essential obstacles. If HMOs were meant to reduce fragmentation in health care systems, how could an HMO development effort be administered as just another categorical HSMHA program and still remain a comprehensive solution to health care delivery system chaos? The organizational limitations of HSMHA were, after all, merely the institutionalization of the shortcomings of the entire health system.

Valiante, in short, forced HEW senior officials to face up to an unpleasant truth: by giving HSMHA lead agency responsibility — however sensible this decision was in terms of the organization chart — they had, in effect, mandated that HMO would be managed as just another categorical grant program. At least for this first round, HEW could not have both innovation and speedy output, not if existing grant authorities and procedures were the mechanism for implementation.

Riso came to these realizations during the months of conflict, in the spring of 1971:

> I [Riso] . . . became aware of two things: that no one had clearly defined what the implication for the special office downtown was, in giving HSMHA the lead agency operation . . . and Vern [Wilson] was operating on the thesis that the baton had been handed to him. . . .[17]

One way to resolve the conflict would be to organize a permanent HMO office in HSMHA substantially staffed by professionals recruited from outside the agency who possessed a distinctive HMO development perspective. Another resolution would be to expand the authority of the HMO project office downtown.

Wilson secured the appointment of Gordon MacLeod, M.D., as director of the HMO development program. By allowing him to appoint his own HMO director, Richardson and Veneman, in effect, settled the controversy between the HMO project office and HSMHA in HSMHA's favor. It had taken over eight months to settle this dispute.

In September, Riso left the Office of the Secretary to become the HSMHA Associate Administrator for Resource Development.[18] The

---

17. Gerald Riso, interview, Dec. 1973.
18. MacLeod told Wilson that under no circumstances would he take the job of HMO director to serve as a physician "front" for the real "HMO czar," Gerald Riso. A

HMO project office in HSMHA would report to him, but he would not directly administer the program. As Riso put it, "I went out there simply because I felt that they needed somebody with an implementation attitude to get this thing on the road and to stop this eternal bickering between Valiante and Wilson."[19]

When Riso arrived on the job at HSMHA in September 1971, he realized "for the first time that John was raising damn legitimate questions." Valiante's main complaint, after the grants were let in June, was that the grantees were the same establishment groups — doctors, hospital-based grantees. Riso verified this for himself when he arrived at HSMHA. His criticism was biting:

> You don't have a good geographic mix. You don't have a good mix of sponsors. All you are going to do is prove that a bunch of white physicians operating in a well-to-do community can provide medical care for people who have money without proving a damn thing about HMO in one way or the other. More specifically, I didn't see any specific program objectives in mind.[19]

Myers, who was chiefly responsible for the first grant round, disagreed with Riso's assessment:

> We wanted to get a balance among regions. We wanted to get a balance between rural and urban, between provider, consumer, and hospital sponsorship. We tried to get a balance among the various kinds given the limited amount of money we had. And to a certain extent I think we achieved that pretty well. We had at least one grant in each region and a pretty good balance.[20]

The argument was moot to the extent that the Secretary's staff perceived the results of the first grant round negatively; and, in any event, a new team to plan subsequent developmental efforts was being assembled.[21]

---

bargain was, therefore, struck giving Riso coordinating responsibility for HSMHA's five development programs (CHP, RMP, NCHSRD, Hill-Burton, and HMO). MacLeod believed that with Riso's authority encompassing all of these programs, he would be left reasonably alone to manage the HMO program.

19. Gerald Riso, interview, Dec. 1973.
20. Beverlee Myers, interview, July 1974.
21. To be sure, the new team was being brought on board during the spring of 1971, one by one. Frank Seubold, Ph.D., from the West Coast aerospace industry, arrived in May; William McLeod, from Booz-Allen-Hamilton, came in as a consultant in March; and Gordon MacLeod, M.D., who had begun his consultation in February, became *de facto* HMO director in July, *de jure* in December.

The Second Grant Round: An Exercise in Strategic Planning

The newly installed HMO management group, led by Riso and MacLeod, sought to accomplish three objectives in planning for the second grant round, to be funded in December: to achieve a better geographic mix; to balance out perceived distortions in the types of organizations that received awards by finding grantees not already committed to the HMO concept but interested in sponsoring one, or converting to the HMO format; and, finally, to set up a two-stage funding process replacing the single, lump-sum award.

The idea behind the two-stage funding process was that the federal government could interest physicians, community groups, and hospitals in exploring the feasibility of getting into the HMO business before either they or the government committed substantial resources to the development process. These "feasibility awards" would amount to $25,000 each. Only some awardees were expected to get through the feasibility process into the second stage, "Development." But, of those selected after the feasibility stage to receive large ($100,000-500,000) development awards, a significant number were expected to reach full operations. By the time these grantees reached the end of the development phase, new legislation was expected to subsidize initial operating losses through a program of loans and loan guarantees. This phased approach to the use of the feasibility and development funds, then, assumed that a third phase of funding (which would require legislation) would be available, beginning in mid-1972, for loans and loan guarantees. In all, 70 projects were supported in December 1971, using only 314(e) funding and reflecting the new management team's attempts to balance out first-round sponsorship distortions. The two-stage approach of committing the bulk of awards in small feasibility studies was implemented and only a relatively small number of large, development grants were awarded.

The Two Grant Rounds in Perspective

It is difficult to discern any noticeable change in the distributions of grants among regions and across project types in the December round, when the new management team was in place, in comparison to the hastily constructed earlier grant round in June 1971. Of course, as Riso noted, the plan was to phase in newer priorities over the course of a number of rounds. Unfortunately, from Riso's viewpoint, the work was incomplete at the end of the second round.

Certain trends were discernible. The regional distributions remained about the same, but there were shifts made in December among sponsor types. Foundations for medical care and insurance companies/private organizations were reduced in December, while physician groups, hospitals, and medical schools were significantly increased. Consumer group sponsorship remained level. In other words, traditional sponsors of HMOs were being deemphasized in favor of reaching out to medical care organizations not usually identified as HMO sponsors. The program was reaching out beyond the insular HMO family to non-HMO-oriented health care organizations, a policy necessitated by the ambitious reforms yet to be accomplished, but fraught with danger and unknown consequences.

Congress Kills the Third Grant Round

Planning for a third round of grants that would complete one full fiscal year of funding commenced even as final funding decisions were being completed for the second round. The burden of fully supporting the HMO effort out of 314(e) funds was being volubly protested by the Community Health Service, which managed the 314(e) comprehensive health services projects. As an alternative, the use of Section 910(c) funds (Regional Medical Programs) was again suggested as an appropriate vehicle, and the Assistant General Counsel once more supported the concept.[22] A concerted effort to improve sponsor-type distributions beyond the corrections already made in the second round was a central feature of the forthcoming round.

In January, 97 contract proposals for new HMO planning and development projects were received. These were solicited from the HSMHA regional offices, which evaluated the applications for technical quality. Then, central office staff sorted them out according to type of sponsor. It was decided to fund 40 of the applications seeking a good sponsor-type balance across regions.

The funding never happened. At the end of February, Sen. Edward M. Kennedy (D-MA) and Rep. Paul G. Rogers (D-FL), chairmen, respectively, of Senate and House health subcommittees, sent a joint letter to Richardson, requesting that he halt further development of HMOs pending passage of enabling legislation that would provide the Administration with specific guidance as to congressional intentions for the structuring of such an effort. The legislators were deeply concerned about the Administration's aggressive development of HMOs in the absence of

---

22. Sidney Edelman, "Funding Sources for HMO Projects," memorandum from the Assistant General Counsel for Public Health to the Director HMOS, HEW/Office of the Secretary, Dec. 16, 1971. Section 910(c) funds, however, were available for planning purposes only. RMP funds could not be used to support operational HMOs.

explicit congressional guidance. They were bothered by the spectre of a large number of HMOs created through the Administration's (questionable in their eyes) use of reprogrammed funds from other PHS authorities. Because the Congress was well into the shaping of its own HMO program, it found the Administration's behavior intolerable. Not only was HEW tapping monies from categorical programs funded for other purposes, but also it was usurping congressional prerogatives by shaping its own HMO program without regard to Congress.[23]

During the last week in February, Richardson told his Assistant Secretary for Health, Merlin K. DuVal, to halt the upcoming third grant round, scheduled for funding in April 1972. DuVal passed the bad news to Wilson, Riso, and MacLeod at a meeting, ostensibly called to discuss MacLeod's and Riso's request for release of funds to carry on the third round of awards. Paradoxically, Riso had only recently increased his projections as to the number of new starts the Health Maintenance Organization Service (HMOS) could handle.[24]

> DuVal simply announced that, after consultation with the Secretary, that was the end of all grants to new grantees. DuVal simply announced it to us at the meeting with no discussion, really . . . and DuVal simply announced that he and the Secretary had decided.[25]

Wilson was forced to take the unpleasant and embarrassing step of sending out letters to each of the 97 applicants that no funds would be available to them. The letter did leave the door open to technical assistance, however, since the Secretary's order was to halt new planning and development, but said nothing about nonmonetary (technical) assistance or the continuing support of present grantees.

The reaction of the HMOS team was predictable: they were shocked. Riso and MacLeod sent a memo to Wilson expressing their dismay with the Assistant Secretary's decision:

> The immediate cessation of any additional HMO planning and developmental activities during this fiscal year raises a serious ques-

---

23. The Secretary had stated on a number of occasions that HEW's goal was to fund 450 HMOs by FY 1976 and 1,800 by FY 1980. These estimates were somewhat lower than the 1,700 HMOs originally promised by FY 1977. While legislation was anticipated to support this effort, it was clear from the rhetoric that HEW viewed legislative support as an augmentation of its own efforts.
24. In October 1971, the HMO offices had been formally reconstituted as the Health Maintenance Organization Service (HMOS). Gordon MacLeod, M.D., was formally appointed director in December.
25. Gerald Riso, interview, Dec. 1973.

> tion of credibility for DHEW/HSMHA and the Health Maintenance Organization Service (HMOS) particularly in view of the fact that a review cycle is nearing completion. . . . On the National scene, a serious question on the Administration's credibility to back up the President's commitment in his February 18, 1971, Health Message must be expected. . . . For these reasons, I recommend that the present funding cycle and existing contract activities for technical assistance be brought to a successful conclusion.[26]

MacLeod's request went unheeded, and the April 1972 funding cycle was cancelled. Over the next two months, however, efforts to salvage the HMO development program within the narrow constraints applied by the Congress went forward in the Secretary's office.

The Care and Feeding of Emergent HMOs

Even though the April funding cycle had been cancelled, 79 projects were active from the two previous rounds. Of immediate concern to the HMOS team was the well-being and continuing progress of these projects. Fortunately, there was support for this position in the Office of the Secretary, and, within two months of the cancellation of the April grant round, over $18 million of funds had been reprogrammed for activities in support of the HMO effort. This unexpected improvement in the HMO program's fortunes must be viewed against the backdrop of the Administration's continuing battle with the Congress over Public Health Service program priorities. For, while Congress was instructing the Administration not to fund any new HMO starts, it was also appropriating $102.7 million for the Regional Medical Program, a $50 million increase over the Administration's request.

Richardson, as tactfully as possible, informed Rep. Daniel J. Flood (D-PA), chairman of the HEW Appropriations Subcommittee, that "We have already announced our intention of obligating the full amount appropriated, but the extra funds require us to make some adjustments in funds budgeted for program management.[27] In other words, the Administration would not impound the increased appropriation but its price would be to use a "portion of this increase to extend support to development of Health Maintenance Organizations. Approximately $16 million is being devoted to this purpose in 1972."

---

26. Gordon MacLeod, M.D., "Funding of HMOS Contracts," memorandum from the Director, HMOS, to the Deputy Administrator for Development, with a "cc" to the Administrator, Feb. 28, 1972.
27. Elliot L. Richardson, letter to Hon. Daniel J. Flood, HEW/Office of the Secretary, Mar. 15, 1972.

In addition, the Secretary informed Flood, "We are planning to reprogram $2.2 million from funds appropriated to the National Center for Health Services Research and Development (Section 304) from 'grants and contracts' to 'direct operations' — and to use these funds in tandem with the Regional Medical Program."

The Section 304 funds would be used to expand substantially the HMOS staff by 116 new positions, the bulk of these to be regional office technical support staff. Richardson was, in essence, broadening his organizational commitment to HMO, even while adhering to the congressional prohibition against funding new HMO projects. Blocked from expanding the absolute number of HMO projects, HEW now sought to enhance its capacity to care and feed what it had already established. Flood's response indicated his displeasure:

> There has been Congressional criticism of the extent to which you have already been engaged in these activities. In view of the foregoing it would be quite presumptuous of me to speak for the Subcommittee.
>
> I intend to call a meeting within the next few days in order to determine the consensus of the Subcommittee concerning this matter.[28]

The HEW Secretary also notified Rogers of his intended use of reprogrammed funds in a similar letter of explanation, sent about a month later:

> As I am sure you are aware, there is clear legislative authority in Section 910 of the RMP legislation for this support, and further affirmation of the legislative authority was contained in last year's Senate Report on the fiscal year 1972 appropriation.[29]

At first, it appeared that Congress would not block HEW's plans. Congressional supporters of HMO were put in a position where they themselves could not appear to be backpedalling on their own HMO commitments. Having forced HEW to stop expanding its program prior to authorization, they could not, only weeks later, signal yet another retrenchment by blocking the Administration's efforts to assist extant programs. There would be little to be gained by such an action, except to

---

28. Daniel J. Flood, M.C., letter to Hon. Elliot Richardson, U.S. House of Representatives/Committee on Appropriations, Mar. 23, 1972.
29. Elliot L. Richardson, letter to Hon. Paul G. Rogers, HEW/Office of the Secretary, Apr. 25, 1972.

give heart to HMO opponents, who were waiting for the right moment to launch an attack on the program.

These negotiations, however, gave the HMOS management team an extremely short time in which to mount a substantial technical assistance program. Of the $16 million available through RMP, they were able to commit $7 million in the space of approximately one month. In addition, about $4 million in grants were committed to continuation of previously funded HMO projects.

The $7 million of reprogrammed RMP funds covered a number of activities. There were, first of all, 10 Technical Assistance Program (TAP) teams, consisting of consulting firms contracting to provide specialized technical assistance to developing HMOs in such areas as actuarial analysis, market determination, and financial planning. In addition, contracts were made with six "resource development organizations" to develop HMO capabilities among their memberships.[30] This device was a rather clever way of indirectly supporting the start of new HMOs without directly controverting the intent of Congress. The idea was that each of these organizations would work with about five of its constituents and help move them toward HMO development. As a result of this program, a few clinics and FMCs converted to HMO status and became operational. These national development organizations represented a diverse mix of health care constituents, and by supporting them, the HMO program, in effect, was furthering its aim of developing a broad base of HMO sponsors. The resource development project never realized its potential, however, because the selected national membership organizations did not (or could not) deliver on their promises.

The enthusiasm engendered by the rebound from the third grant round cancellation was to be short-lived. By the end of the fiscal year 1972 — June 30 — it was clear that the long-awaited legislation needed to relieve HMO of its stepchild status was not going to come before the end of the 92nd Congress.[31] Now Flood's displeasure with the building of a substantial personnel force by reprogramming 304 funds came back to haunt HEW during negotiations with the Health Appropriations Subcommittee. The Secretary was told not to persist in building a work force without specific congressional authority. The HMOS was notified that

---

30. The organizations were: Association of American Medical Clinics, Association of American Medical Colleges, American Association of Foundations for Medical Care, National Medical Association Foundation, Group Health Association of America, and the Medical Group Management Association.
31. Gerald R. Riso, "FY 73 HMO Plans," memorandum to the Administrator, HEW/HSMHA, May 8, 1972.

instead of adding substantial new staff, it would have to reduce its work force drastically. As it turned out, Riso and MacLeod were able to hold most of their permanent staff, but they had to relinquish their consultants, which comprised about half of their total work force:

> From July of 1972 on we were really strapped for people. This was unfortunate because here we had a lot of resources available to use, and yet, we really didn't have the people to manage these things the way they should have been managed.[32]

A *De Facto* Demonstration

An irony of the period of retrenchment characterizing the Administration's HMO development program from July 1972 until the passage of P.L.93-222 in December 1973 was that, by circumstance rather than design, a limited national demonstration program had, in fact, already been carried out with 79 projects over a three-year period. To an extent, then, the complaint from HMO detractors that HMOs were untested had been rendered moot. Beyond the earlier 40 years' experience, there were now three years of active federal experience available for evaluation. As described in the next chapter, congressional staff benefited substantially from this evolving experience through frequent contact with HMOS personnel.

The 1972-73 period of project development and technical assistance provided four critical pieces of information about what kinds of HMO projects would and would not work. First, it was absolutely essential that the sponsoring organization be committed to developing an HMO. Some of the institutions that accepted feasibility grants were not serious about HMO development, viewing it as an educational experience or as another program for getting money out of the "feds." A second element was the importance of involving physicians in the planning of an HMO from the beginning. Some projects, practically ready to become operational, could not, at the eleventh hour, deliver a group of doctors willing to work in the HMO setting. Third, it was important to have an effective executive director. The talent pool for HMO management personnel was rather limited, and some projects were impeded by having directors not up to the task. The fourth critical element was the ability to make a fair estimate of the market potential in the service area. Thus, as time passed, the HMOS team developed a greater sensitivity to the problems to be overcome before a project could become operational.

---

32. Frank Seubold, interview, Feb. 1974.

Pressure on the Right: A National Election Intrudes

Throughout the springtime difficulties with the Congress, the White House had been, for all intents and purposes, silent. Nevertheless, President Richard M. Nixon again reaffirmed his Administration's continued commitment to HMOs in his March 1972 health message to the Congress.[33]

As the race for the Presidency warmed up toward the fall of 1972, the Administration began to reevaluate its HMO posture. Any shift in position was subtle and, perhaps, initially unnoticeable to all but the most discerning of observers. It came as a consequence of growing opposition from the American Medical Association, which had, by mid-1972, become thoroughly alarmed by the progress of HMOs. AMA was exploring ways to restrain the ardor of the Administration and the Congress.

AMA brought strong pressure on the Administration to reduce its commitment to the HMO movement. Malcolm Todd, M.D., a member of the AMA's executive board and Nixon's former physician, personally interceded with the President.[34] AMA's Washington lobby requested that Minority Leader Rep. Gerald R. Ford (R-MI) intercede with Kenneth R. Cole, special assistant to the President, in opposition to HMOs.[35] But what hurt most of all was the departure in 1972 of HEW staff that had long supported HMO: Richardson, Veneman, Butler, Riso, Valiante, Wilson, and, in the spring of 1973, MacLeod.

It was soon clear that the new Secretary, Caspar W. Weinberger, lacked Richardson's enthusiasm for HMOs. MacLeod observed:

> Something happened in the spring [of 1973] that convinced me to be aware that there was now an official follow through. . . . Weinberger had a press conference or meeting and declared that HMO was now a demonstration. . . . Then in June, at a press conference, he declared it was an experiment.[36]

The code words were there to be read and pondered. Until the fall of 1972, the Administration, speaking through Richardson and his staff, had firmly held that HMOs had been well tested over the past 40 years and that they were essential alternatives in health care organization. The Secretary's most conservative development plans had called for HMOs

---

33. Richard M. Nixon, Special Message to the Congress on Health Care, Mar. 2, 1972.
34. John K. Iglehart, Health Report/Intense lobbying drive by medical group dims prospects for HMO legislation. *National J.* 4:1404, Sept. 2, 1972.
35. *Chicago Sun-Times* reports and AMA staff memos. See chapter 6, page 148-149, for a full account of AMA's intercession with Ford.
36. Gordon MacLeod, interview, May 1974.

being available as an option to 90 percent of the populace by fiscal year 1976. This was a major federal commitment to a fully developed effort.

The AMA had steadily chipped away at Richardson's position, privately presenting a variety of arguments about HMO shortcomings, but publicly supporting HMOs as a model of health care organization that required further experimentation and demonstration. A full federal commitment, AMA suggested, not only would be foolhardy, but also would represent an unfair tilt against the nation's fee-for-service solo practitioners.

Weinberger's use of the words *demonstration* and *experiment* were signals of a substantial shift in Administration policy. Moreover, the Administration had revised its HMO development proposal in Congress to reflect this new, scaled-down perspective, calling for a limited experimental program and, most significantly, omitting any reference to preemption of restrictive state laws.

The White House officials most intimately involved with the program readily acknowledged a more sober approach to HMOs in 1973. Deputy Assistant of the President Kenneth R. Cole Jr. portrayed the Administration as caught between a number of advocacies. The Administration remained committed to the HMO concept but had always supported a limited demonstration effort, not an open-ended federal commitment. HEW had, perhaps, been overzealous in its advocacy. According to Cole:

> The position of the Administration, in my mind, has been very clear throughout the whole thing. I don't dispute the fact that the President's instructions were embellished as they came out of HEW . . . most specifically by the Senate, until they got reined in. But the President's instructions starting in December 1971 have been consistent with a demonstration program. . . .[37]

The new 1973 position, then, was merely a reaffirmation of the Administration's commitment to HMOs within the limits of policy constraints to which it had always adhered.

There are three problems with this argument. First, if the 1971 and 1972 HMO commitments were overzealous, then why had the White House consistently let them go unchallenged? Second, the President himself had gone on record in his 1971 health message as supporting HMOs as the cornerstone to his health delivery system reform proposals. He had committed himself to the goal of making HMOs available to 90 percent

---

37. Kenneth R. Cole Jr., interview, Oct. 1974.

of the population within five years. Third, and most specifically, the Administration had totally reversed itself on the issue of preemption of state laws restricting group practices and other prepayment plans.

With the departure of HEW's most articulate and enthusiastic HMO advocates, and Nixon's rightward drift following his impressive 1972 electoral victory, the AMA was finding more willing listeners both at HEW and at the White House. And the spectre of a runaway Senate HMO bill originating from the President's arch rival, Kennedy, had been, in the words of one official, "frightening as hell." It added weight to the arguments of those preaching caution.

The Reorganization of H

The Public Health Service (the H in HEW) was reorganized in 1973, right on schedule. HEW had, in fact, been "reorganized" about every three years since its creation in 1953. The 1973 reorganization reflected the influence of the "management perspective" on the Republican Administration and its use of "functional management principles" as a political instrument in the continuing struggle against categorical programs.

HSMHA and other elements of the PHS were reconstituted into four new agencies: the Health Resources Administration (HRA); the Health Services Administration (HSA); the Center for Disease Control (CDC); and the Alcohol, Drug Abuse, and Mental Health Administration (ADAMHA). This realignment of the components of the PHS was intended to strengthen the control of the Assistant Secretary for Health over health programs and to reduce the number of entities directly reporting to the Secretary.

Another objective of the 1973 reorganization was to decategorize program elements within the bureaucracy. This was to be accomplished by establishing "functional" line divisions within each agency's bureaus and by submerging some of the individual categorical program services to the level of "desks" within some bureaus, particularly in the Bureau of Community Health Services. The net result would be to make such divisions as "policy development," "organization development," and "monitoring and analysis" the preeminent units, replacing heretofore highly visible categorical health programs, such as "maternal and child health," "neighborhood health centers," and, inevitably, "health maintenance organizations." Most significantly, core professional staffs would be distributed among the functional units, leaving only skeletal staffs to hold down the substantive program desks.

To the leadership of the HMOS, submergence to desk status was an indignity that could not go unchallenged. Throughout the spring of 1973,

MacLeod fought to retain the HMOS intact as a viable unit within either HRA or HSA. But he could not prevail and resigned in July 1973, protesting the action as "another attempt by the Administration to disregard the intent of Congress, which has proposed legislation to demonstrate HMO as an alternative health care delivery system."[38]

On July 1, the HMOS was disbanded and its nearly 100 employees either distributed among other (functional) divisions or terminated (many staffers had been hired on temporary status or as consultants). The "HMO desk" consisted of a holding action group of about six people, headed by Frank Seubold, Ph.D., who had served as chief of the management division in the now defunct HMOS. The HMO desk had virtually no operating budget and could make no new allocations. Of the 79 original projects, 25 "had gone down the drain." "This was no real surprise, since the expected financial support for initial operating deficits never materialized. But on the other hand, 16 or so had managed to get into full-scale operation. . . ."[39]

Legislation was the key. Without it, the HMO program would be finally and irrevocably disbanded. By September, legislation seemed, at last, to be a virtual certainty. It had taken nearly three years for Congress to complete its work. Why had it taken so long?

---

38. Gordon K. MacLeod, M.D., Announcement of Resignation from Directorship of HMOS, July 1973.
39. Frank Seubold, interviews, Jan. 1974 and Jan. 1979.

CHAPTER 5

The Legislative Struggle: Part I

By the summer of 1973, the Administration had been implementing a growing HMO development program for more than two years, under the dubious charter of prior congressional authorizations. Although a specific legislative direction had become critical, such a mandate was not easily forthcoming. This chapter explores the reasons for congressional tardiness in passing HMO legislation.

The Setting: Congressional Health Committees and Subcommittees

The Congress reduces complex health issues to specifically focused elements, which are assigned to separate subcommittees, each jealous of its own legislative turf. Although this procedure allows individual legislators to concentrate on important details, the particularity of the subcommittee system also fragments issues and works against comprehensive solutions. Committee rivalries and overlapping jurisdictions tend to exacerbate procedural problems.

HMO was a particularly vexing issue because it combined, in one comprehensive set of organizational innovations, both the payment for health services and the plans for their organization and delivery. Since its earliest ventures in support of personal health services, Congress had carefully observed the distinction between "payment" and "services delivery." The distinction both reflected and reinforced underlying practices in the private health sector, where paying for existing services by the health insurance industry was an entirely separate enterprise from those activities that produced health resources and delivered health services.

Public payment for health services has been guided by the philosophy and perspective of the Social Security Act (42 USC §301 *et seq.*), while resource development and service delivery programs have been guided by the Public Health Service Act (42 USC §201 *et seq.*). The Social Security perspective is different from the health services and resource development perspective. Both have acquired their own unique world views, their own constituencies, and their own notables. These perspectives persist, inside and outside the federal government, in both the executive and legislative branches, crosscutting and often confounding labels such as Republican and Democratic, liberal and conservative.

Federal health service payment programs emerge from Titles V, XVIII, and XIX of the Social Security Act. Title V authorizes formula grants to states and special project grants to public and nonprofit organizations to provide maternal and child health and crippled children services to mothers and children eligible for welfare support under other titles of the law. Title XVIII, Medicare, is essentially a health insurance program for retirees, while Title XIX, Medicaid, provides payments through state programs for certain medical services to eligible categories of welfare recipients. Both Medicare and Medicaid, incorporated in the Social Security Act, are financed through a combination of employer-employee payroll taxes. And tax policy jurisdiction falls to the House Ways and Means Committee and to the Senate Finance Committee.

These two committees recruit from like-minded constituencies. They are well stocked with bankers, businessmen, and corporate and tax lawyers ever watchful about guarding the interests of the private sector against grandiose public-sector schemes. The Senate Finance Committee plays a guardianship role, serving as the oversight committee for the Social Security trust funds. It perceives its task to be that of prudently managing the trust funds and guarding against policies that might expose them to fraud or extravagance. Since 1966, Medicare and Medicaid had turned out to be exorbitant in both respects. Hence, the committee was in the midst of a general reappraisal of these programs when first confronted with the HMO proposal during the summer of 1970.

In Jay Constantine, then as now, an influential staff aide responsible for health legislation, the guardianship role of the Senate Finance Committee has found a staunch and most able steward. Outraged by the runaway costs of Medicare and Medicaid, Constantine took the lead in researching and writing a startling legislative report (published in

February 1970) that thoroughly documented these escalating costs.[1] Constantine believed that the government should maintain a tight rein on persons and entities spending federal taxpayers' money and, more specifically, on disbursements from the Social Security trust funds. He sought, with increasing vigor in 1970, to prod the Social Security Administration's staff — especially Robert Ball, Arthur Hess, and Irwin Wolkstein, key managers of the Medicare program in the early 1970s — to monitor the health provider community more effectively.

* * *

In contrast to health services payment, health resource development and service delivery programs focus on the federal role in shaping or altering the nation's supply of health resources and methods by which the health care system delivers its services. There are two key full congressional committees and their corresponding subcommittees that share responsibilities for health resource development and service delivery legislation.

On the House side, there is the Interstate and Foreign Commerce Committee and its Subcommittee on Health and the Environment. The committee handles health affairs almost as an afterthought, along with commerce, communications, transportation, and utilities, deriving its jurisdiction over health as a result of its responsibilities for tariffs and the Merchant Marine (the Public Health Service hospital system). The Subcommittee on Health and the Environment has jurisdiction over such matters as drug abuse, health professional education, cancer research and development, and water and sanitation programs.

On the Senate side, the Labor and Public Welfare Committee (now renamed the Committee on Labor and Human Resources) has jurisdiction over health, labor, and welfare legislation. This committee is usually packed with liberals from both the Democratic and Republican parties. Historically, it has enthusiastically sponsored large-scale social programs. Its Subcommittee on Health and Scientific Research is an aggressive body, usually taking a liberal approach to health policy. Sen. Edward M. Kennedy (D-MA) has been the chairman since 1971 and a leader in seeking to improve the health care delivery system. Kennedy could usually rely on a unified subcommittee, with even liberal

---

1. See: "Medicare and Medicaid: Problems, Issues, and Alternatives," Report of the Staff to the Committee on Finance, U.S. Senate, Feb. 9, 1970.

Republicans like Jacob K. Javits (R-NY) and Richard S. Schweiker (R-PA) supporting his positions. In the early 1970s, there was one major dissenter on this subcommittee, conservative Sen. Peter Dominick (R-CO).

The House and Senate Search for Cost Containment Strategies

The Administration was not the only branch of government searching for a national health policy in 1969 and 1970. The Congress also was trying (as it still is) to deal with the problem of escalating Medicare and Medicaid costs. The Senate Finance Committee commissioned the previously mentioned staff study to analyze issues and alternative solutions to skyrocketing health care delivery costs under Titles XVIII and XIX. The committee began its intensive investigation in 1969, held a brief hearing in July, and published the detailed report on February 9, 1970.[2] In the interim, the committee received testimony from hundreds of witnesses, who related horror stories of how the Medicare and Medicaid programs were being abused by participating health care providers, especially physicians, hospitals, and "welfare mill" clinics. In its final report, the Senate Finance Committee offered reams of statistics that documented excessive and unnecessary utilization of health services under Titles XVIII and XIX. The report concluded that before reimbursing providers, closer scrutiny must be given to the content of their services.

Meanwhile, on the House side, the Ways and Means Committee began holding public and executive sessions in the fall of 1969 (continuing into 1970) on possible legislation to improve the operating effectiveness and efficiency of the Medicare, Medicaid, and Maternal and Child Health programs. Against this backdrop of congressional hearings and investigations into health cost containment, the Administration introduced its Part C HMO option in late March 1970. The House Ways and Means Committee served as the appropriate forum for Under Secretary John G. Veneman to present the Administration's health maintenance strategy on March 23. As it happened, the committee's executive sessions on welfare reform proposals and Social Security amendments were wrapping up,

---

2. The Administration's own search for national health policy was spurred, at least in part, by pressures from the Senate Finance Committee. In July 1969, Under Secretary Veneman had been pointedly called to account for the chaotic state of the Medicaid program during hearings of the Finance Committee. See chapter 1, p. 8. The Finance Committee resumed these hearings in February and asked Administration officials to respond specifically to the criticisms of Medicare and Medicaid raised in the report of the Finance Committee staff. See: Medicare and Medicaid, hearings before the Committee on Finance, U.S. Senate, Feb. 25 and 26, 1970, Part I.

and Veneman was working almost continuously with the members.[3] The Part C option would have authorized the Secretary of HEW to implement prospective rates of payment on an experimental basis to hospitals and extended care facilities for services rendered to Medicare and Medicaid clients. It was a modest proposal.

Words such as *gradual, selective,* and *experimental* ran throughout the proposed amendment. Only a limited patient population was to be included in this experiment (Titles XVIII and XIX beneficiaries), and it restricted the types of health care providers eligible to participate. Chairman Wilbur Mills raised no serious objections, and the task for the Administration was to translate Part C into legislative language suitable for insertion into H.R.17550, the omnibus Social Security Amendments of 1970. Between the end of March and the beginning of May, a legislative proposal was drafted.

Ways and Means: Hospitable to HMOs

The House Ways and Means Committee spent the better part of March, April, and May of 1970 marking up the complex bill H.R.17550. The HMO proposal did not surface again until May, when the Administration formally offered its HMO proposal to the committee in legislative form. The final HMO proposal met with little resistance in the Ways and Means Committee, which found the Administration's proposal timely, as well as ideologically and politically hospitable on three counts.

First, the HMO proposal was introduced when Congress was eager to develop strategies to stop rising federal health care expenditures. Second, the proposal did not upset the prevalent private-market orientation of the committee, because it provided for purely financial incentives to be tacked onto the health care delivery system and did not attempt to modify directly the organizational components of that system. Third, the HMO concept was politically acceptable because it called for no additional financing from the beleaguered Social Security trust funds. It was, quite simply, a limited innovation that might produce significant cost savings in the future. The Ways and Means Committee reported out H.R.17550 and published its final report on May 14.

The rationale for instituting a prospective reimbursement policy mirrored the Administration's call for modifications of federal health services payments under Medicare:

---

3. For a description of how the Administration made its presentation, see chapter 2, pp. 42-43.

> [Your] Committee believes that payment determined on a prospective basis offers the promise of encouraging institutional policy makers and managers, through positive financial incentives, as well as the risk of possible loss inherent in that method, to plan, innovate, and generally to manage effectively in order to achieve greater financial reward for the provider as well as a lower total cost to the programs involved.[4]

Further, the Ways and Means Committee agreed with the Administration's prudent approach to authorizing small experimental and demonstration projects. This was consistent with the sound business practice of committing small amounts of money to an innovative idea and to evaluating the results. If the policy initiative failed, then little would be lost; if it succeeded, more projects would be authorized for further expenditures. The committee wrote:

> In view of the far-reaching implications of such a change in the approach to reimbursement, [your] committee's bill provides for a period of experimentation under Titles XVIII, XIX, and V with various alternative methods and techniques of prospective reimbursement. It is the intent of [your] committee that experimentation be conducted with a view of developing and evaluating methods and techniques that will stimulate providers through positive financial incentives to use their facilities and personnel more efficiently, thereby reducing their own as well as program costs while maintaining or enhancing the quality of the health care provided.[5]

The language of the House version of the HMO proposal reflected the willingness of the Ways and Means Committee to offer HMOs a flexible reimbursement mechanism within which to prove their worth. The language was very general: the Secretary of HEW was authorized to offer HMOs "a combined Part A and Part B, prospective, per capita rate of payment for services provided for enrollees in such organizations. . . ."[6] The rate of payment would be determined annually by taking into account the HMO's premium experiences with other (non-Medicare) enrollees, allowing for differences in utilization between these younger enrollees and Medicare-eligible (older) enrollees. The payment, however, could not exceed "95 percentum of the amount that the Secretary es-

---

4. U.S. House of Representatives, "Social Security Amendments of 1970: Report of the Committee on Ways and Means on H.R.17550," House Report No. 91-1096, May 14, 1970, p. 29.
5. *Ibid.*, p. 30.
6. *Ibid.*, p. 116.

timates . . . would be payable for services if such services were to be furnished by other than health maintenance organizations."[7]

On May 21, 1970, H.R.17550 passed the House of Representatives. In only three months, the health maintenance concept had moved from an informal discussion at the Dupont Plaza Hotel in February 1970 to a full legislative program passed by one house of Congress. However, in the months to follow, the Senate Finance Committee would slow progress on HMO policy. HMOs were to arouse deep-rooted suspicions among the fiscally conservative membership and staff of the Finance Committee. At a time when the committee was recommending its own cost containment proposals in the Constantine report, which called for greater regulatory oversight in the Medicare/Medicaid reimbursement systems, the HMO proposal called for prospective reimbursement, a method of payment that would make increased monitoring of provider services much more difficult. Or, so the Senate Finance Committee came to believe. The HMO proposal was in deep trouble in the Senate.

Trouble in the Senate Finance Committee

The Finance Committee received the bill in early June 1970. The key staff person voicing immediate skepticism was Jay Constantine. He noted that the committee's approach to Medicare reform was not to abandon fee-for-service payments, as proposed by the HMO option, but to advocate stricter regulatory controls and monitoring of fee-for-service reimbursement, a course of action consistent with the committee's oversight responsibilities. Prospective reimbursement, at a predetermined, fixed price, the heart of the HMO proposal, ran directly counter to this approach and would substitute the self-control of market incentives for the regulatory policing of the Social Security Administration and its mentor, the Senate Finance Committee. HMOs were indeed alien to the Social Security perspective.

Not surprisingly, Medicare program staff in the Bureau of Health Insurance of the Social Security Administration also criticized the HMO option that emerged from the House. BHI routines were designed to reimburse the costs and fees of hospitals and providers, not to advance payments without regard to the actual costs and amounts of provided services. The euphemistic phrase *prospective reimbursement* did not make the language in the House version of H.R.17550 any more palatable. Where were the controls? What if an HMO's cost experiences were less

---

7. *Ibid.*, p. 116-117.

than 95 percent? Should the HMO then get to keep all of the savings? Would this not be an inequitable subsidization of HMOs from the Medicare trust fund by non-HMO Medicare (Part A and Part B) subscribers? Sound accounting principles, as well as equity, required that the BHI review an HMO's cost experiences after services had been rendered and make some kind of adjustment.

Thus, the market incentive principle came into direct conflict with the protectionist ethos of the Social Security system, both in the bureaucracy and in the Senate Finance Committee. Anticipating a hospitable forum in the forthcoming Senate Finance Committee deliberations, the Social Security Administration began to reshape the HMO payment formula presented in the House bill. Characteristically, the first concern of Social Security staff was with the precise meaning of the term *prospective reimbursement.* "The question is whether the rates so determined prospectively are final or interim rates. Can they be adjusted retroactively based on actual experience?"[8] This question was artfully phrased. By raising it, the Deputy Chief Actuary of the BHI was, in essence, asking for clarification of the relationship between initial payment (based on estimated HMO premium experience) and actual cost. The whole issue of retroactive adjustments to payment could then be raised. The question, in short, emerged from Social Security's experience in advancing payments to Part A providers (hospitals), with the understanding that periodic adjustments based on actual cost would be made. The basis of the prospective payment to an HMO was its permanence based on price. It was meant to be a firm price, a budget that had to be kept. Any retroactive adjustment worked directly counter to the incentive for cost efficiency at the heart of the prospective reimbursement concept.

Social Security staff was also concerned with the issue of "retention." "In calculating the capitation rates, what should be the retention factor that SSA allows in addition to the actual costs of providing services?"[9] The House had been purposely silent on this matter, accepting the Administration's argument that the public's interest was well served by the 95 percent ceiling on reimbursement. If an HMO could deliver services for less, then its reward for efficiency was retention of the difference between its actual expenses and the 95 percent reimbursement rate.

The Finance Committee, however, would be receptive to acceptance of the 95 percent payment rate only if it were tied to a strict formula limiting

---

8. William C. Hsiao, "Payment Formula for Health Maintenance Organizations," memorandum to Chief Actuary,.Social Security Administration, May 20, 1970.
9. *Ibid.*

retention. In other words, it wanted a delineation of precisely how much an HMO could retain (of savings, if costs were below the 95 percent reimbursement rate) and what such retained earnings had to be used for. Such specificity went well beyond what even the supercautious Social Security staff was advocating. Thomas Tierney, the Medicare staff director, related Constantine's stance to a colleague in late June:

> Jay Constantine called me Friday to talk about HMOs. . . . He . . . [suggested] that a limitation should be set on the retention rate of any participating HMO. He suggested that the retention percentage for over 65ers should not exceed the retention percentage for under-65ers, or that the dollar amount of retention for those over 65 not exceed 150 percent of the dollar amount of retention for those under 65. I told him we would give some thought to appropriate retention limitations, but that there would be strong support from HIBAC* and elsewhere for the idea that the 95 percent figure be a floor rather than a ceiling, in which case there would be no necessity for computing an allowable retention. *Jay's reaction to this approach was very negative* [emphasis added].[10]

Constantine believed that the HMO proposal, as presented by the House, was tantamount to "having the government write out a blank check" to health care providers. He was concerned about letting "the marketplace roam on its own" without any type of legislative control. Moreover, some health care providers would render less care than was required in order to stay within their prospective budget constraints.[11]

The Senate Finance Committee began public hearings into H.R.17550 on June 11, 1970. Private negotiations between the Administration, represented by Social Security and HEW secretarial staff, and the Finance Committee staff continued through the summer and into the fall. It was clear that holding the line with the flexible House version would be completely untenable. Therefore, Secretary Elliot L. Richardson's project group reluctantly accepted Social Security's position calling for retroactive adjustment of the 95 percent rate of reimbursement.

In early October, the staff report incorporating the draft language for the HMO provision of H.R.17550 was published. In his cover memo conveying the Finance Committee staff recommendations to Veneman,

---

*The Health Insurance Benefits Advisory Council.

10. Thomas Tierney, Notes on a telephone conversation with Jay Constantine, Social Security Administration, Bureau of Health Insurance, June 22, 1970.
11. Jay Constantine, interview, June 1974.

Social Security Commissioner Robert Ball noted that HEW had gone into negotiations with a number of suggestions for improving the House bill. These were accepted, however, only after Finance Committee staff "received assurances that we would accept . . . a number of changes insisted upon by Mr. [Tom] Vail [General Counsel] and Mr. Constantine." Deputy Commissioner Hess noted in a separate memorandum to the Under Secretary that:

> Despite our efforts to dissuade them, Finance Committee staff have insisted, as you know, on writing into the "Blue Book" that the committee will have before it when it considers the HMO proposal certain limitations on the amount of retention that will be recognized in computing the HMO's adjusted premium for Medicare enrollees. . . . We hold no brief for such a limitation, but we have been completely unsuccessful in our efforts to convince the Committee staff to eliminate or liberalize it.[12]

The Finance Committee staff report (the "Blue Book") criticized the House version and suggested improvements. The main thrust of the recommended changes was the modification of prospective reimbursement and retention, but other changes were proposed as well. The staff left no doubt, however, that the thrust of these changes was to ensure that HMO's darker side could not victimize either the Medicare trust fund or enrollees.

The Finance Committee stipulations were strong medicine indeed. They were certainly not designed to encourage substantial conversion of Medicare contracts to the HMO model. The Administration had hoped to dissuade the Finance Committee staff from its inflexible approach — at least with regard to retention. However, Hess reminded his HEW colleagues of "the extremely hazardous prospect" of raising "any objections in Executive Session to the Senate Staff's retention provision . . . when we were trying to finish all the pending business this week." Once the mark-up copy had been conveyed by staff to the full committee, the Administration's leverage was effectively lost. If the Administration could not work its will with staff, it would find no sympathy with the senators themselves.

Some thought was given to an Administration lobbying effort to get a more favorable HMO bill out of the Senate or out of a House-Senate conference. But the calendar was working against HMO prospects in the

---

12. Arthur E. Hess, Limitations on HMO Retention, memorandum to the Under Secretary, Social Security Administration, Oct. 16, 1970.

91st Congress. Because the Finance Committee had combined President Richard M. Nixon's controversial Family Assistance Plan (welfare reform) proposal and a foreign trade proposal with the Social Security Amendments of H.R.17550, the bill ran afoul of a filibuster during the last two weeks of December. By the time welfare reform and foreign trade proposals were belatedly dropped, it was already December 29 — time enough to pass H.R.17550 by a vote of 65 to 25, but no time for a conference with the House. H.R.17550, therefore, died at the end of the 91st Congress.

H.R.1 and the Containment of HMO

When the Senate Finance Committee combined consideration of welfare reform with Social Security Amendments toward the end of the 91st Congress, it ensured against early passage of an HMO Medicare measure in the 92nd Congress. Even the most cynical congressional observer, however, would not have predicted that it would take nearly two years, until October 1972, to get the HMO measure out. The HMO Medicare proposal became captive both to the fortunes of welfare reform and to the intense scrutiny of skeptical Senate Finance Committee staff.

The President had placed his full prestige behind the HMO concept, however, by making it a principal component of his national health strategy on February 18, 1971. Recognizing that he could not rely solely on the outcome of protracted debate in the Ways and Means and Finance Committees, the President broadened the HMO initiative to include a comprehensive development program that would require unique authorizations and appropriations from general revenues. Where Congress was concerned, it made sense to hedge one's bets by having more than one legislative option available. The alternative HMO development proposal would engage the efforts of House and Senate Health Subcommittees, shifting the legislative arena to the Public Health Service Act, and away from the Social Security Act.

Meanwhile, the HMO Medicare proposal continued its unsteady course through the congressional Social Security committees. H.R.1 was introduced in January 1971 by Chairman Wilbur Mills and referred to his Ways and Means Committee. The HMO provision (Section 239) was identical to the one passed by the House the year before. Over the next two months, Social Security Administration staff persuaded a generally responsive Ways and Means Committee staff to accept a number of modifications, which were adopted during executive sessions. Among them was a clarification of the basis for determining the estimated 95 percent prospective payment. The problem identified by Medicare staff was the excessively complex actuarial analyses that would be required to establish the "premium-related equivalent" (non-HMO rate) upon which the 95 percent prospective rate would be based.

Social Security staff proposed, and Ways and Means accepted, a simplified method for determining actuarial premium equivalence. It was a variation of the "community rating" concept, based on establishing geographical area average rates, rather than the more complex "experience-rating" approach, which required comparisons among particular demographic segments of a population. By allowing HMOs to establish their prospective rate in comparison with average area costs for Medicare beneficiaries not enrolled in an HMO, the actuarial analysis problem would be greatly simplified.

A second area in which the Ways and Means Committee accepted modifications was to include language requiring control of retention. The House bill had been silent on this matter in the previous session, but the stringent formula included in the Senate version required a response. Ways and Means, however, adopted a provision for control of retention that was far more flexible than that adopted by the Senate Finance Committee in the previous session:

> To guard against potentially excessive profits from the Medicare payment, your committee has included a provision to assure that the rate of retention (gross revenue less costs) for Medicare enrollees would not be permitted to exceed the rate for other beneficiaries of the health maintenance organization. Since an acceptable rate of retention cannot be prospectively assured, the provision calls for an examination by the Secretary of the actual rates of retention experienced by the organization. . . . Any report showing a positive rate of retention for Medicare enrollees which exceeds 90 percent of its rate for other enrollees would be subject to full audit. Where an excessive rate of retention is verified, the organization would be required to utilize such excess for additional benefits or reductions in premiums charged to Medicare beneficiaries or to refund the excess to the trust funds.
>
> For purposes of this provision, an "excessive rate of retention" would ordinarily be any positive rate of retention for Medicare enrollees which exceeds the organization's rate of retention for enrollees under age 65.[13]

13. U.S. House of Representatives, "Social Security Amendments of 1971, Report of the Committee on Ways and Means on H.R.1," House Report No. 92-231, May 26, 1971, pp. 90-91.

These provisions demonstrated the willingness of Ways and Means to address the problem of potential abuses, if no controls were instituted, while allowing sufficient flexibility in the amount and use of retention to maintain the incentive features of cost efficiency. H.R.1, including the HMO Medicare proposal, was favorably reported to the House of Representatives on May 26, 1971, and was passed one month later. As in the previous Congress, the Senate Finance Committee would have the last word.

It soon became clear that Finance Committee staff, guided by Constantine, would again subject the HMO Medicare proposal presented by the House to intense critical scrutiny. A clue to the direction of Constantine's thinking came in the form of a detailed list of questions presented to HEW in late July 1971.[14] HEW's response arrived in mid-September. The questions required HEW to make highly specific responses regarding Administration views on HMO organization, quality of care, and cost considerations. A number of questions, in particular, requested clarification of the nature of reimbursement mechanisms and retention provisions proposed in H.R.1.

Finance Committee staff, unconvinced of the wisdom of the Administration-backed HMO provisions in H.R.1, set out to develop its own provisions for reimbursement and retention. By early 1972, the staff had developed proposals that went well beyond those developed during the previous session for the Senate version of H.R.17550.[15] These new proposals virtually abandoned the prospective reimbursement concept altogether and severely limited the rate of retention allowable to an HMO. Constantine and his colleagues were still determined to bring the HMO concept into substantial conformance with already established Medicare reimbursement procedures.

"Established" HMOs — those that had demonstrated at least three years of successful operating experience — would be eligible for capitated incentive reimbursement payments, payable in fixed monthly installments, based on an operating cost and enrollment forecast presented to HEW by the HMO. This interim reimbursement rate would be adjusted quarterly to reflect any changes experienced during the year, and HEW's payments would be adjusted accordingly. Thus, the 95 percent prospec-

---

14. U.S. Senate, Committee on Finance, Health Maintenance Organizations, staff questions with responses of the Department of Health, Education, and Welfare, Sept. 27, 1971.
15. See: "Report of the Committee on Finance to accompany H.R.1, The Social Security Amendments of 1972," U.S. Senate, S. Report 92-1230, 1972, pp. 229-244.

tive rate had been abandoned in favor of this interim cost-reimbursement mechanism. The Finance Committee staff genuinely believed that since the payment was to be allocated to the HMO in advance of actual service provision in a lump sum, it represented a substantial accommodation by the Medicare program to the usual method of reimbursing an HMO.

At the year's end, the HMO's adjusted average per capita cost would be calculated. This figure would be the hypothetical cost that would have been incurred to provide services for the HMO-enrolled Medicare recipients under conventional fee-for-service arrangements and in other HMOs. At the same time, the HMO would report its actual costs. Then, the final reimbursement to the HMO would be calculated. If the HMO's costs were less than 100 percent of the adjusted average per capita cost, the savings would be shared between the HMO and the federal government. Savings of up to 10 percent of the adjusted average per capita cost would be divided equally between the government and the HMO. The next 10 percent of savings (if any were realized) would be divided 75 percent to the government and 25 percent to HMO. And savings greater than 20 percent, if there were any, would go entirely to the government. The HMO could earn savings or pass them on to beneficiaries. Losses would also be shared in similar fashion: to be carried forward and fully recovered from savings. But government losses would be recovered before future savings would be paid to an HMO. This proposal came to be known as the "savings-sharing, loss-sharing" formula.

The Finance Committee recommended, however, special treatment for new HMOs with less than two years' operating experience. They would be reimbursed on a cost-only basis. The Secretary of HEW would contract with developing HMOs for an interim periodic payment, which could be adjusted "at the end of the contract period to reflect the HMO's expenses otherwise reimbursable under Title XVIII of providing covered services to its Medicare enrollees."[16]

These proposals to reimburse established HMOs on an at-risk basis (providing some incentive for cost-efficiency by allowing fractional retention of savings) and new HMOs on a cost-only basis both departed significantly from the flat, fixed-sum prospective premium approach advocated by the Administration and the House. In both instances, the Senate Finance Committee staff was proposing variations of a retroactive rate adjustment based on costs.

---

16. *Ibid.*, p. 236.

The sharpest criticism of the Senate Finance Committee provisions came from Paul Ellwood, who had been serving as an HEW consultant during this period, working with the HMO Project Office. His critique came in the form of a letter to Sen. Russell B. Long (D-LA), chairman of the Finance Committee. Ellwood called attention to the fact that the basis of the HMO policy was the fixed-price contract established in advance:

> In our opinion, it is the HMO policy which will eventually bring us true value for money rather than piecemeal attempts at containing overspending in the present disorganized system. . . . [The technical formulas] proposed by the Committee to limit any potentially excessive earnings by HMOs . . . begin with the retroactive determination of HMO costs. Any such cost determination immediately violates the incentive principle inherent in price reimbursement and essentially returns us to cost reimbursement. Because of the long-term incentive effects, cost reimbursement cannot be cheaper than price reimbursement, even though the price may contain some earnings. Contrary to price reimbursement, providers paid by cost have every incentive to increase cost and thereby cash flow. There is no way in practice to effectively police the multitudinous ways by which costs can inflate in the practice of a field as complex and professionalized as medicine.[17]

The way to ensure against HMOs delivering less service for a fixed price or service of a lower quality, noted Ellwood, would be to monitor the provision of services. He endorsed his own proposal for the formation of a new federal regulatory commission to monitor health outcomes as the best means to monitor the value of service.[18] He also recommended that the Finance Committee reconsider its own position and accept the

---

17. Paul M. Ellwood Jr., M.D., letter to Sen. Russell Long, Apr. 6, 1972.
18. The Health Outcomes Commission proposal was first presented by Ellwood at a conference on health care quality assurance, sponsored by the American Rehabilitation Foundation, in New Orleans, in January 1972. Subsequently, Sen. Edward M. Kennedy adopted this approach to quality assurance in his HMO bill, S.3327. However, the Senate Finance Committee adopted the Professional Standards Review Organization (PSRO) approach, which emphasized its preoccupation with use of regulatory procedures to control the costs of health care. Ellwood believed the Finance Committee's preoccupation with cost regulation rather than with return on medical service value (that is, the results or outcomes of medical care) was in error. See: Paul M. Ellwood Jr., M.D., and others, Assuring the Quality of Health Care, Minneapolis, MN: InterStudy 1973, for a full discussion of the quality assurance issue as it relates to HMOs.

language of the House-passed version of H.R.1 with regard to prospective payment.

Ellwood's letter had no impact on the Senate Finance Committee's position. In fact, one Social Security staff member suggested that his criticism could have a negative impact on Finance Committee staff, who might

> tend to be resentful of what they will consider an erroneous statement . . . [that] the committee's proposal is simply cost reimbursement, without incentives to lower costs or to form profitable HMOs.

Then, reflecting the Social Security Administration's inherent caution in its delicate relations with Senate Finance Committee staff, the Medicare program staff member noted that HEW would

> continue to try to make changes in the provisions the committee has in mind to advance us toward the goals we have in mind. The places where we are most likely to be effective with obtaining such changes are on the Senate floor and in conference. We'll have to be careful in any case not to upset the applecart, however, by insisting on more than is enactable.

Protracted executive sessions, principally on welfare reform provisions in H.R.1, took up most of the Senate Finance Committee's time between April and September 1972. Staff recommendations on the HMO provisions were accepted without debate. The bill was reported to the Senate on September 26, 1972, with just three weeks remaining in the second session of the 92nd Congress. Nine days of heated, sometimes acrimonious, debate over the welfare reform provisions immediately followed, and the bill passed the Senate on October 6, only after all welfare reform proposals had been deleted. H.R.1 went to conference with only 10 days remaining in the second session.

The House-Senate conference had less than two weeks to reconcile differences in a bill over 900 pages long (even after the controversial welfare reform proposals had been deleted). Long stood firm behind his staff's work on HMOs, and the House acceded to the Senate on all of its amendments, with two exceptions.

First, Ways and Means conferees succeeded in getting Senate conferees to accept a simplified version of their savings-sharing formula, as recommended by HEW HMO staff. Thus, in place of the Finance Committee's three-tiered savings-sharing formula (up to 10 percent, the next 10 percent, over 20 percent), House conferees substituted a simplified formula: "Savings up to 20 percent of the adjusted average per capita cost shall be apportioned equally between such organization and the Medicare Trust Fund."[19] Savings over 20 percent would revert entirely to the trust fund. In other words, up to 20 percent of realized savings over costs would be split 50-50 between the HMO and the trust fund.

Second, Ways and Means conferees were also successful in deleting the loss-sharing features for established HMOs. Thus, an HMO would be at risk for costs incurred above average adjusted per capita costs. This feature was all that could be salvaged from the original House provision for a flat 95 percent (of average area per capita costs) prospective reimbursement rate.

P.L.92-603, the Social Security Amendments of 1972, was signed by President Nixon on October 30, 1972. Section 226 (1876, in the Social Security Act) provided for reimbursement of HMOs in the two ways essentially proposed by the Senate Finance Committee, with slight modifications by the House. Established HMOs would receive a payment based on their annual average adjusted per capita costs plus a portion of savings as retention. New HMOs would be reimbursed on an actual allowable cost basis. Neither provision bore much resemblance to the prospective, fixed-price reimbursement feature originally embodied in the Nixon Administration's Part C HMO proposal and substantially retained in the House-passed version of H.R.1. The Senate Finance Committee had converted that proposal into a thinly disguised version of the cost reimbursement methods already employed in reimbursing conventional carriers under Part A of Title XVIII.

Final promulgation of regulations implementing Section 1876 did not come until late in 1976. The complex nature of these provisions and their precise meaning were the subject of protracted discussion among Social Security and Senate Finance Committee staff. No established or new HMOs could avail themselves of the provisions of the law until the regulations were published. Nor did the final promulgation of regulations engender great enthusiasm in the HMO community. Expected administrative difficulties with Section 1876 of Title XVIII acted as a powerful disincentive to participation in the program.

By early 1979, only one reimbursement agreement had been entered into between BHI and an HMO under the at-risk (savings-sharing) prospective reimbursement formula. Several HMOs, however, had elected to undertake Medicare contracts under the full-cost reimbursement

---

19. U.S. House of Representatives, "Conference Report to Accompany H.R.1," 92nd Congress, Second Session, House Report No. 92-1605, Oct. 14, 1972, p. 16.

mechanism. Given the nature of the elderly service population and the lack of incentives to balance the risks, it is little wonder that those few HMOs that have cared to participate in the program at all prefer the security of full-cost reimbursement guaranteed retroactively.

The Senate Finance Committee had done its work all too well. In its zealous effort to guard the Medicare trust fund, it had effectively neutralized the HMO Medicare option. By 1978, only about 25,000 Medicare-eligible older Americans were enrolled in HMOs. Efforts to modify the reimbursement method were sporadically attempted. Not until 1978, however, did a promising new departure appear imminent. The Carter Administration, reacting to the virtual absence of any appreciable enrollment of Medicare-eligible populations in HMOs, submitted fresh proposals to the Ways and Means and Finance Committees. Constantine had been right about one important element: a 95 percent fixed rate of reimbursement clearly would represent a windfall profit to most HMOs, given the dramatic inflation of the mid-1970s. In fact, the one at-risk contract that could be reviewed, with the Health Cooperative of Puget Sound, indicated that actual cost experiences were substantially below the 95 percent rate. By early June 1978, HEW officials had refined their proposal to revise the Medicare HMO reimbursement formula. It called for HMOs to be reimbursed prospectively on the basis of an adjusted community rate. If this rate exceeded 100 percent of the average adjusted per capita costs (AAPCC) for all providers, the HMO could elect reimbursement under an alternative method, which, essentially, would allow the HMO to charge premiums for deductibles and coinsurance, excluding retention. However, this alternative would only be available for up to three years if the HMO's costs exceeded 100 percent of the AAPCC.

The Administration's HMO Development Bill: A Broadened Initiative

Advocates for HMO realized in 1971, no less than in 1978, that any hope for vigorous federal promotion and development of HMOs, would have to come about through a whole new HMO development program under the Public Health Service Act. The Social Security Act, although it had the greatest long-term potential for driving the whole health system toward cost efficiency, was years away from fundamental reform. The Administration's commitment to HMO, therefore, led to the launching of an aggressive development program, administered under existing authorizations in the Public Health Service Act. The political and operational hazards of implementing such an initiative without specific authorization and budget, however, impelled HEW planners to design legislation for explicit development of HMO projects in order to secure and protect their embryonic program.

Clearly, the HMO Medicare amendment was an inappropriate vehicle for the development of new HMOs. For one thing, the bureaucracy responsible for the development of new HMOs — the Health Services and Mental Health Administration — had absolutely no claim on the Social Security budget supporting Medicare and its own bureaucracy, BHI.[20] Furthermore, the Medicare trust fund could not be utilized for substantial resource capitalization. Among the HMO amendments that passed the 92nd Congress, Section 222 did provide for experimentation and demonstration of incentive reimbursement arrangements, but it clearly did not envision the wholesale conversion of health system components into HMO configurations. Moreover, Social Security Administration staff doubted whether these incentive reimbursement provisions could even be applied to HMOs now that these organizations had their own unique authority under Section 1876 of the Social Security Act.

On February 18, 1971, therefore, when Nixon delivered his national health strategy message, he broadened his HMO initiative beyond the Social Security (Medicare) proposal and promised to reorganize the health care delivery system by using federal money directly to stimulate development of HMOs. As part of this effort, the President promised to submit appropriate legislation to Congress. On March 4, 1971, the Administration's first HMO development bill, H.R.5615, was introduced by Rep. Harley O. Staggers (D-WV), chairman of the Committee on Interstate and Foreign Commerce; and on March 10, 1971, the Senate version, S.1182, was introduced by Jacob Javits, ranking Republican member on the Committee on Labor and Public Welfare.

The Administration's proposal would authorize the Secretary of HEW to make grants to or contracts with public or not-for-profit HMOs, and contracts with profit-making HMOs, to develop new HMOs or expand the operations of functioning HMOs. The Administration's bill also provided for loan guarantees for profit-making HMOs to establish themselves, to provide new or expanded health services, and to offset their initial operating losses. The Secretary could make direct loans to public HMOs to meet initial operating costs incurred in medically underserved areas. Loan guarantees would be limited to construction of outpatient or ambulatory care facilities or to operating costs for not more than three years. The bill also created an HMO Loan Guarantee and Loan Fund.

---

20. In fact, the record shows that, through most of the 1970-73 period, communications between the two bureaucracies were infrequent.

H.R.5615 reflected the Administration's desire for a flexible approach to HMO development. The bill was purposely general in specifying types of organizational entities that could qualify as HMOs and the range of services they would have to offer. Six conditions were established. The entity must: (1) provide service on a per capita prepaid basis; (2) provide or arrange for a prescribed range of services; (3) provide physicians' services, whether by employment, contract, or arrangement with groups or individual practice organizations, on a fixed-price prepaid basis; (4) demonstrate financial and operational competence; (5) ensure access, prompt services, and quality, and (6) have open enrollment under certain conditions.

H.R.5615 responded to Nixon's call for an HMO-based national health strategy in all major respects save one: the bill omitted any reference to the problem of restrictive state laws and the need for federal authority to override them if they precluded HMOs. However, in subsequent congressional testimony, Administration officials supported the preemption concept.[21]

The Administration was walking a fine line between the predisposition of federal law and regulation to indicate highly specific uses for public funds and the requisites of the HMO approach, requiring flexible investment capital, at some risk, to stimulate innovation in the health care market. The focus of the Administration, or at least of the HMO Project Office in the HEW Office of the Secretary, was clearly to design the simplest possible investment program in keeping with federal statutory limitations. The health industry, after all, needed proper incentives and gentle guidance from the federal government to restructure itself. So the Administration's bill took great pains to encourage private, for-profit entities to participate in the development program. The strategic use of the terms *public, private,* and *nonprofit* conveyed clear messages to the thoughtful reader. To plan and develop HMOs, public and nonprofit private organizations could apply for grants, while for-profit entities could undertake contracts. Similarly, loans to offset initial operating losses would be available only to public and nonprofit entities but profit-

---

21. HEW Secretary Richardson favored a two-stage strategy: (1) of developing a model state law favorable to HMOs (which states could then adopt), and (2) of exercising the preemption requirement in contracts between HMOs and Medicare and Medicaid. In other words, the Secretary opted to cover the preemption issue through amendment of health insurance provisions, rather than under an HMO assistance act. Elliot L. Richardson, "Decision Issue: What Should We Do about State Legal Barriers to the Formation of HMOs?" HEW, Feb. 1, 1971.

making HMOs could avail themselves of federal loan guarantees.

The project manager for HMOs in the Office of the Secretary, however, felt that H.R.5615, as drafted, was too limiting, especially to public entities. The bill should provide for below market interest rate loans to public HMOs and utilization of a loan "take-out" procedure similar to that used by the Federal National Mortgage Association (FNMA). He objected also to the provision limiting loans to public HMOs covering only costs of operating in underserved areas. This would not permit public HMOs "to overcome . . . their larger problem of modernization of facilities or construction of ambulatory care facilities." The solution would be to "expand the direct loan authority to cover hospital modernization and ambulatory care facilities regardless of service area."[22]

These criticisms raised important prior questions: for what, through what mechanism, for how much, and for how long would the federal government subsidize HMO development? Public Health Service staff assumed the legitimacy of special subsidies to health underserved areas. But weren't there other justifications for such subsidies? And wasn't the awarding of grants or contracts in itself a form of special subsidy for a particular mode of medical practice? The federal government had never before ventured this far in expressing a preference for a particular form of health care delivery for the mainstream of the populace. Prior investments in neighborhood health centers, after all, were limited to specialized populations, for example, the poor, infants, and so forth.

H.R.5615 also called for an annual open-enrollment period. The problem with such a provision, according to the HMO Project Office critique, was that it unfairly burdened HMOs with enrollment responsibilities not required of voluntary and indemnity health insurance plans. This requirement was intended to prevent unscrupulous HMOs from skimming off enrollees with fewer health problems in order to reduce operating costs. However, commercial insurers and even Blue Cross Plans, in effect, engage in skimming when they use their actual experience with specific groups to establish preferential premium rates for some and less favorable rates for others.

These issues were not immediately resolved, but they provided an early indication that to draft an acceptable HMO development law would be a complex and time-consuming job. As the number of individuals and

22. John D. Valiante, "Current Inadequacies of HMO Act," memorandum to the Under Secretary and Deputy Under Secretary, HEW, Office of the Secretary, Apr. 1, 1971.

groups participating in that process broadened, the range of issues and opinions would also expand.

From the outset, neither the House nor Senate health subcommittees showed much enthusiasm for the Administration's HMO development bill. Their negative reactions were, in part, reflexive responses of congressional Democrats to executive branch Republicans. Beyond that, it was clear that the Nixon Administration had gone well beyond traditional Republican approaches in staking out its HMO policy. Thus, many traditional, fiscally conservative Republicans reacted more negatively to the HMO proposal than did the Democrats. The ensuing conflicts ran deeper than party cleavage and were interwoven with a number of institutional issues as well as issues unique to health affairs. These conflicts gradually crystallized as the Senate and Health subcommittees, in their own time, came to consider the HMO approach seriously.

The House Democratic Counterproposal: Rep. Roy's Initiative

When the 92nd Congress convened in January 1971, newly elected Rep. William R. Roy (D-KS) was offered a place on the health subcommittee. His selection was hardly surprising: Roy was both a physician and an attorney. More remarkable, perhaps, was the fact that, although he had been elected vice-speaker of the Kansas Medical Society House of Delegates in 1970, he was actively opposed in his election bid by the Kansas Medical Political Action Committee (KAMPAC). Nevertheless, KAMPAC efforts to the contrary notwithstanding, Roy engineered a startling upset over his long-time incumbent, conservative, Republican opponent.

In late May, Roy offered his services to House health subcommittee chairman Paul G. Rogers (D-FL) in tackling an important piece of health legislation that might be pending before the subcommittee. Roy was eager to develop a unique and visible position in health affairs, in no small part because his reelection bid in the normally Republican second district of Kansas would require him to move on health issues, a promise he had made to his constituents.

Rogers, for his part, was interested in protecting Democratic votes on his subcommittee, as well as in the House. Therefore, he took the unusual step of not only offering Roy the opportunity to take a look at "something called HMOs, a bill that the Administration put in, in March," but also promising to cosponsor a new bill with Roy.[23] This

23. Brian Biles, M.D., interview, June 1974.

would likely ensure the bill's favorable reporting to the full Committee on Interstate and Foreign Commerce. Rogers took this action because, while a Democratic response to the Administration's HMO bill, H.R.5615, was called for, his calendar was full of more pressing commitments for the remainder of 1971.

Shortly after receiving Rogers's permission to draft a House response to the Administration's HMO bill, Roy asked the AMA's Washington-based Democratic lobbyist for help in drafting it. This lobbyist was eager to overcome the bad feelings between Roy and the AMA, caused by KAMPAC's failure to support his election bid. He promptly arranged a meeting with technical experts from the AMA's Chicago headquarters; but, greatly to his embarrassment, the headquarters staff turned Roy down, asserting that its constituents could never support a bill of that type.

Roy was outraged by the AMA response. He had considered himself a loyal member and officer of AMA's Kansas component, and he was genuinely puzzled by this second rebuff in less than a year. It was the last time the congressman sought help from the AMA, and, paradoxically, AMA, by this action, denied itself a golden opportunity to influence the shaping of the House version of HMO legislation.

Roy and his young staff aide, Brian Biles, M.D., a newly graduated physician from the University of Kansas, sought information and help in other, more hospitable quarters. They began at the Group Health Association of America (GHAA) conference in Washington, DC, in June 1971.[24] There they had the first of many discussions with GHAA officials, who told them, then, that H.R.5615 was a "very broad and general bill."[25]

From June 1971 to November 1971, Biles worked tirelessly to write a comprehensive HMO bill that would speak to the ambiguities of the Administration's proposal. He spoke to many people, primarily technicians who were both policy analysts and administrators, academicians who were either economists or medical care administration specialists, and members of health interest groups. Biles's purpose, during this period, was to build an HMO statute taking full advantage of the breadth of experience and knowledge of these HMO professionals.

He came to rely on a small, inner circle of advisers, who could react to revisions and alternatives that emerged as conversations with HMO

24. GHAA is the national organization representing prepaid group practice plans.
25. Brian Biles, interview, June 1974.

technicians increased in frequency. Significantly, Ellwood and his staff broadened their own involvement, after the President's February 1971 message, to include the congressional committees. Biles particularly valued the judgments of Rick Carlson and Patrick O'Donoghue, M.D., of Ellwood's staff, who made frequent visits to Washington as HMO advocates and technical consultants. Thus, even as the circle of actors involved in HMO policy making expanded to include a wide assortment of health interests, Ellwood, the original proponent of HMOs to the Nixon Administration, found himself close to the center of efforts to construct a congressional Democratic alternative.

As Biles's inquiries moved forward, a core of significant deficiencies in the Administration's bill, H.R.5615, came into focus. In Biles's own words:

> It [H.R.5615] was too vague. [I] read the bill and didn't know what they were going to do. They were talking about groups that led me to be concerned about the problems of skimming and skimping. Are they really groups which are not going to provide comprehensive care? . . . were not going to have open enrollment? . . . were not going to have consumer participation . . . ?[26]

Biles personally believed that the Administration intentionally produced an ambiguous bill to give the profit-making sector an incentive to enter the HMO development market and to give a Republican Administration maximum flexibility to implement a program compatible with its free market ideology. Referring to the Administration's proposal, Biles said, "It was clearly profit oriented."[27] Because the Administration did not state specific group-practice arrangements and loosely defined the benefit package, Biles realized that

> what we are not going to get now are new Kaisers and new Puget Sounds; we are going to get a lot of new foundations and a lot of for-profit groups. . . .
>
> We had a track record of 20 years and millions of people who had been participating in prepaid groups. What have we learned? . . . So we talked to people and found that there were a number of features [of H.R.5615] that people were pleased with and other features that people were not pleased with. So, we tried to write legislation work-

26. *Ibid.*
27. *Ibid.* Biles's reading of the Administration's intentions was quite accurate: Certainly, the bill was intended to provide a broad and flexible framework for all manner of organizations to qualify as HMOs.

> ing with a mandate of desirable features [while] prohibiting the undesirable features.[28]

By early November, Roy and Biles were ready with their draft bill, and on November 11, 1971, the proposal was introduced by Roy and Rogers and assigned to the health and environment subcommittee as H.R.11728. Roy announced that day on the House floor that his bill "takes a much more expansive view of the federal role in developing HMOs than does the Nixon Administration."[29] H.R.11728, as one Washington political observer put it, "attempted to deal with provisions in the Administration's proposal that Roy regarded as inadequate."[30]

It reflected a genuine attempt by the congressman and his aide to specifically address complex issues and concerns raised in their consultations with the health community. H.R.11728 reflected another, more subtle departure as well. Unlike the Administration's bill, the Democratic alternative emerged from a belief that government must provide detailed and specific guidance to the health community about acceptable or unacceptable behavior. The idea that the health care marketplace could be trusted to respond (or was capable of responding), in a socially responsible way, to highly general and flexible federal guidance was considered naive.

The congressman and his aide were reacting, in their bill, to a legitimate concern with congressional prerogatives, a distrust of the Nixon Administration's intentions, and a responsiveness to the range of opinion and advice they had received from the health community:

> . . . The issue [was] not whether HMOs are clearly defined. . . . We [saw] the issue as who is going to make the decision? We have seen legislation written before we got here that was essentially three lines long. It said the Administration could do anything it wanted to. This was a period where you had John Ehrlichman saying, "The hell with the Congress." They were proposing legislation that was five sentences, which said, "Here is a lot of money. The Administration can do anything it wants to with it."[31]

---

28. *Ibid.* NOTE: Biles's reference to "Kaisers" and "Puget Sounds" was to two of the oldest and most prestigious nonprofit group practice HMO plans. "Foundations" referenced "Foundations for Medical Care," loose confederations of solo practice physicians, usually spun off from a county medical society, to provide a fixed benefit package of services, either prepaid or fee-for-service.
29. *Congressional Record,* Nov. 11, 1971.
30. John Iglehart. Health report: Democrats cool to Nixon's health proposal, offer their own alternatives. *Nat. J.* 3:231, Nov. 20, 1971, p. 231.
31. Brian Biles, interview, June 1974.

H.R.11728 differed from the Administration's HMO bill in five key ways. First, it defined HMOs in highly specific language, including the types and amounts of services that had to be provided. Second, the bill presented specific dollar amounts for planning, development, and initial operation of an HMO.[32] Third, it recognized only public and nonprofit organizational entities; there was no provision for participation of profit-making HMOs in the benefits of the law. Fourth, the bill mandated a role for consumers in HMO policy making, including grievance procedures. And fifth, the bill provided for an override of state laws that restricted the formation or operation of HMOs. There were also quality assurance provisions, requirements for open enrollment, community rating, and health education for both subscribers and staff.

HMO Project Office staff in HEW's Office of the Secretary summarized its reaction to H.R.11728 as follows:

> [H.R.11728] is similar to our bill in that it provides a variety of types of support (grants, contracts, loans, interest subsidies, and loan guarantees). It is better than our bill in that it contains a legal barrier override. And it is worse than our bill in that it requires an HMO to provide a too comprehensive benefit package, precludes any for-profit support even for loan guarantees, and requires all funding (approximately $750 million in FY '74) to be approved by a 12-man advisory council.[33]
>
> . . . The bill would restrict federal assistance to a rather narrowly defined group of organizations. Most existing prototypes would be unable to qualify for assistance because of requirements for more extensive benefits than currently provided, consumer involvement in policy development, a limited definition of a medical group, mandated emphasis on underserved areas, and nonprofit sponsorship. Foundation plans [individual practice associations] would be excluded, and insurance-underwritten plans such as Harvard and Columbia would be ineligible.[34]

---

32. The Administration had used a similar formulation in its second grant round in early 1972, by providing very small ($25,000) early feasibility planning grants, before committing a larger amount for initial development. H.R.11728, however, would offer up to $250,000 for the planning stage. The Administration was unwilling to commit such a large sum of money to organizations that had not undergone a "feasibility planning" stage, prior to commencing "program development." Nor did they include specific authorization levels. H.R.11728, however, was willing to risk a much larger amount at the planning stage. See chapter 4, p. 77.
33. John D. Valiante, "Several Comments on HMO Legislation Status," memorandum to the Under Secretary, HEW, Office of the Secretary, Nov. 19, 1971.
34. John D. Valiante, "Analysis of Roy Bill on HMO Assistance," memorandum to the Departmental HMO Coordinator, HEW, Office of the Secretary, Dec. 7, 1971.

The critique concluded by noting the administrative complexity created by the bill's provisions with language such as "provided by the Secretary in regulations." The bill reflected little understanding of the problems of managing existing development programs.

The HEW Project Office's criticisms of Roy's bill forecast a number of future trends in all subsequent congressional approaches to the HMO matter: a tendency toward highly specific and broad service requirements; a decided preference for expanding the missions of HMOs beyond those traditionally accepted by extant HMO prototypes (HMOs were now to be instruments of federally inspired health care reform and would have to take on expanded service roles and enrollment responsibilities); and, finally, an unwillingness to define the organizational configurations that would qualify as HMOs in anything but highly specific terms.

Following the November filing of the Roy-Rogers bill, as it came to be known, no further actions were taken until April 1972, when Rogers was able to schedule hearings. Meanwhile, Sen. Edward M. Kennedy had been gradually turning from a frustrating and abortive attempt to stimulate Senate interest in national health insurance to the issue of HMOs.

The Senate Democratic Counterproposal: A Comprehensive Prescription for Change

Shortly after Roy began to craft his own piece of HMO legislation, Kennedy opened hearings on a number of HMO bills. Kennedy's interest in any proposal from the Nixon Administration could only be characterized as unenthusiastic. The senator from Massachusetts was aware of the antipathy and fear in which he was regarded by the Nixon White House: because of his potential role in the 1972 Presidential campaign and also because, more than any other national political leader, Kennedy had come to represent the interests and perspectives of the most liberal of health care reformers. Also, he had not forgotten that the Administration's national health strategy, with HMO as a principal element, had been touted as the Administration's response to his own, labor-inspired Health Security Program. Kennedy and his staff regarded the Nixon Administration's HMO proposal as specifically designed to draw attention away from their own ambitious Health Security Program.

In his years as a junior member of the Senate Labor and Public Welfare Committee, and in his two years of work with the United Auto Workers-sponsored Committee for National Health Insurance, Kennedy had developed an ambitious — some would say radical

— agenda for health service reform. The key was "Health Security," a program envisioning the gradual transformation of the American health system into a somewhat modified version of the British National Health Service, under the aegis of a centralized National Health Security Board. Kennedy was interested in a comprehensive reorganization of the American health services system, in order to make available through aggressive federal actions a full complement of health care services to all Americans, as a matter of public right.

The senator was aware, however, that his ambitious program for health care reform had to confront the realities of the Senate committee system; that, while most of the reforms proposed in the Health Security Program could be considered by his own health subcommittee, the critical financing provisions — the "insurance" aspects — fell within the purview of the more conservative Senate Finance Committee. At precisely the same time that the Finance Committee was considering ways to control Medicare-Medicaid costs, and its staff had reported how health care providers had abused those programs, a number of NHI proposals were referred to the Finance Committee for consideration. Kennedy, however, and his (soon to depart) mentor Sen. Ralph W. Yarborough (D-TX), began their own series of hearings on NHI on September 23, 1970. The move was not lost on Chairman Long of the Finance Committee. But, preoccupied with a loaded calendar of hearings on both Medicare and Medicaid abuses that extended through June, and simultaneously holding hearings on H.R.17550, the Social Security Amendments of 1970, he could not turn to the NHI bills piling up on the Finance Committee's docket, until the spring of 1971. Meanwhile, Yarborough and Kennedy had, by December 1970, concluded their own set of NHI hearings under questionable jurisdictional authority.[35]

---

35. S.4279, the Health Security Act of 1970, was introduced in late August 1970 by Sen. Kennedy to the Committee on Labor and Public Welfare. On September 8, the Committee Chairman, Sen. Ralph Yarborough, introduced S.4328, a slightly amended version of the Kennedy bill, that is, it was funded only from general revenues and not from a combination of general revenues and payroll taxes. Yarborough's move was for no other purpose than to give him an excuse to call hearings on national health insurance. By removing the payroll tax provision, he was artfully able to bypass Russell Long's conservative Finance Committee.
In contrast, Sen. Jacob Javits (R-NY) introduced his own health insurance bill, The National Health Insurance and Health Services Improvement Act of 1970, directly with the Finance Committee. Javits, in remarks before Labor and Public Welfare noted as tactfully as possible that "other" committees besides the health subcommittee had a legitimate interest in NHI.

Both the Javits and Kennedy NHI proposals included strong endorsements of prepaid health care plans. Javits called such plans *comprehensive health service systems,* whereas Kennedy adopted the term *comprehensive health service organization.* Essentially, both concepts were compatible with the Administration's own evolving concept of HMOs, except that, as in the House, the Senate proposals were limited to prepaid group practice plans.

The 91st Congress ended with no definitive Senate action on NHI. Yarborough, defeated in the Texas Democratic primary by Lloyd M. Bentsen Jr., did not return to the Senate and, in January 1971, Kennedy ascended to the chairmanship of the Health Subcommittee on Labor and Public Welfare. He promptly reintroduced S.3, the Health Security Act of 1971. This time, however, Kennedy was unable to repeat Yarborough's strategy of deleting the payroll tax provisions so that the bill could be referred to Labor and Public Welfare, rather than to Finance. Long indicated in strong terms that his committee would not be bypassed in considering NHI.[36] The jurisdictional matter could no longer be finessed. Long prevailed, and Kennedy lost control of his own NHI bill.

When Long finally called his own set of NHI hearings to order on April 26, 1971, it was clear that the concept of national health insurance was in for tough scrutiny by the conservative and cost-conscious Finance Committee. Kennedy himself was subjected to rather aggressive challenges when he testified in support of his bill. In Long's citadel of fiscal conservatism, the central issues of health care delivery reform might easily be lost, as the Finance Committee focused most of its attention on program costs and the need for adequate cost controls, so that the errors of Medicare and Medicaid would not be repeated. In short, the focus of the Finance Committee was more on details of costs, the impact of programs on the Social Security trust funds, and tax burdens on the public. Kennedy's and Yarborough's earlier hearings reflected an entirely different emphasis: on the need to use the financing mechanism of an NHI program as leverage to restructure the health care delivery system.[37]

Long struck a cautious tone when he opened the Finance Committee's hearings on April 26:

---

36. James Doherty, interview, June 1974.
37. Unlike the Nixon Administration's evolving national health strategy, the Health Security Program spelled out, in great detail, the health system structures that needed to be encouraged — namely, prepaid group practice plans. Moreover, in contrast to Republican reliance on the competitive forces of the marketplace to assert cost controls, the Health Security Program had no similar faith. Thus, it called for a single, federally financed insurance system and a rigorously enforced system of price controls.

> Our experience with the enormous cost overruns and administrative difficulties with Medicare and Medicaid justifies caution — to say the least. . . .
>
> We are now turning to the consideration of proposals — some far larger than Medicare in terms of benefits, population covered, and costs.
>
> In large measure, these uncontrolled, rapid rises in health care costs have generated much of the impetus for national health insurance by pricing many people out of the private insurance market and substantially increasing their out-of-pocket costs not covered by insurance.
>
> Substantial success in moderating the costs of health care might very well relieve pressure to the point where a partial selective health insurance program might be more desirable to the American people than the total approach of a national health program.
>
> As a matter of fact, national health insurance itself poses a political paradox. Americans want the best health care money can buy. On the other hand, Americans are predictably sensitive when it comes to paying taxes required to finance this program. No one knows the maximum tax load the American people will tolerate.[38]

Kennedy's testimony sought, artfully, to respond to Long's concerns by showing how the problem of costs was inextricably linked to the malfunctioning of health system components directly resulting from the irrationality of financing methods.

> . . . At every turn, it is financing that causes or contributes to the health crisis.
>
> Because hospital charges are covered by insurance, more people are hospitalized than necessary. Because specialists are reim-

---

Health Security, in short, looked to prepaid group practice plans as a preferred element of a reorganized health care system. The Administration, in contrast, looked to health maintenance as the catalyst for triggering natural competitive market forces. Under Health Security, changes would come about because the government mandated it. Under the Health Maintenance Plan, change would come about because HMOs would prove to be competitively more attractive options. Health Security was a "whole" of which HMOs could be an integral "part." The Health Maintenance Plan promised that, because of HMOs, the "part" would be sufficient enough to reform the entire health care system. Thus, the Administration's own NHI bill, S.1623, was not meant to do more than fill gaps in extant private coverage. The Administration's focus was on HMOs, not on NHI.

38. Russell Long, Opening Statement, National Health Insurance Hearings before the Committee on Finance, U.S. Senate, 92nd Congress, First Session, Apr. 26, 1971.

> bursed at higher rates and enjoy shorter working hours, doctors enter specialties and abandon general practice. Because suburban America can better pay for specialists, doctors flock to the suburbs, and leave rural and urban America to the brutality of hospital emergency rooms. . . .
>
> I am convinced that the way we finance health has trapped Americans in this inefficient and enormously expensive system. My bill, the Health Security Act, aims at breaking open this trap by changing the way we finance health care.[39]

The Senate Finance Committee's hearings ended inconclusively two days later, on April 28, with Long stating, with no apparent feeling of urgency, that "We will go into this matter in greater depth at a later date."

As matters stood in the spring of 1971, then, Kennedy had done about all he could for the Health Security Program. He had even sought to portray the urgency of the health crisis by holding dramatic, but largely ineffectual, hearings entitled "The Health Crisis in America." Barnstorming around the country, Kennedy documented the horrors and abuses the health care system heaped upon the poor, elderly, minorities, and ordinary citizens in general. Lacking jurisdictional authority, however, he could only watch helplessly as Health Security was literally buried among seven other NHI proposals, each representing the views of a different health interest group.

While the health crisis hearings occupied the health subcommittee's time for over four months, an interesting opportunity was developing in the form of a collection of health services delivery reform proposals routinely assigned for possible action to the subcommittee. The Administration had submitted S.1182, its HMO proposal, on March 10, 1971. This bill was identical to H.R.5615, submitted one week earlier in the House. Unlike the situation in the House, however, senators on the health subcommittee had been busy, since 1970, crafting a number of delivery system reform proposals. By July 20, 1971, when Kennedy brought his first set of HMO hearings to order, four other bills, each with an explicit HMO provision or with some other provision synonymous with HMO, had collected on the table. There was, in addition to S.1182, S.935, Kennedy's own omnibus bill "to increase and expand the national

---

39. Edward M. Kennedy, Statement in Support of S.3, the Health Security Act of 1971, National Health Insurance Hearings before the Committee on Finance, U.S. Senate, 92nd Congress, First Session, April 26, 1971, p. 28.

resources for the education of doctors of medicine and osteopathy; and to promote the role of academic medical centers in improving the delivery of health services and medical care." The bill had been developed in consultation with the Association of American Medical Colleges; HMOs were included in the bill almost as an afterthought.

S.935 would expand medical resources through support of medical schools and offered grants "to assist academic health centers in planning and initiating Health Maintenance Organizations." A third feature was assistance "in the establishment and operation of Area Health Education Centers."[40] This initial venture by Kennedy and his staff into the realm of HMO development was significant because it indicated that, as early as February 1971 (when the bill was introduced), they viewed HMOs as only one element of a broader array of health service reforms that focused on substantial expansion and redeployment of the nation's health care resources. From the outset, Kennedy undertook an HMO initiative with expansive reform agendas in mind. In the months to come, as the potentialities of HMO as a framework for large-scale reform became apparent, his HMO initiative would expand even further.

There was one essential difference between the Senate and House health subcommittees' approaches to HMOs: Roy approached HMO as an opportunity to undertake incremental reforms of the existing health system, a perspective not dissimilar in intent from the Administration's, if somewhat more ambitious. Kennedy, however, saw HMO as an expeditious framework through which to pursue his own expansive ideas for comprehensive health care reform.

The Health Security Program, thus, could be pursued pragmatically under the rubric of the Senate version of HMO legislation. And, because the precise meaning of the term *HMO* was highly fluid, it offered an opportunity to develop specific legislation to restructure health care in America. At least in the context of HMO, Kennedy chose to play the radical reformer, while Roy took a more cautious approach. The Administration, of course, found itself playing a more familiar conservative role. All three positions, however, dramatically challenged the status quo of organized medicine.

* * *

40. The concept of Area Health Education Centers was adapted from a 1970 Carnegie Commission recommendation to create a network of centers in order to combat the sense of professional isolation felt by health professionals practicing in rural areas.

Kennedy held extensive hearings on HMOs during the fall of 1971, concluding them in the spring of 1972. In the midst of these hearings, on March 13, 1972, he introduced his own revised HMO bill, S.3327, which replaced S.935 and became the basis fór all further HMO deliberations in the Senate.

The omnibus nature of S.3327 tended to cloud the really important new ingredients that Kennedy and his aide, Philip Caper, M.D., had added to the increasingly complex congressional debate over HMOs. Title III, establishing Area Health Education and Service Centers, was intended to tie area health education centers to federally assisted rural HMOs as part of an overall program of continuing education. Title V was added because many of the categorical program authorities, for example, Hill Burton, Regional Medical Programs, would soon expire and the HMO bill offered a convenient vehicle in which to put these reauthorizations forward.

The key features of S.3327, however, were to be found in Titles I, II, III, and IV. The bill had been ingeniously crafted by Caper so that all its components logically complemented one another. Given the underlying premises of the proposal, S.3327 made much sense.

Title I defined an HMO very narrowly as a "medical group" operating under fixed premium prepayment, which would deliver 12 basic services to enrollees. Title II recognized the restrictiveness of Title I's requirements by creating a new organizational entity, "Health Service Organizations (HSOs)," for rural and nonmetropolitan areas. HSOs did not have to meet the stringent organizational requirements of an HMO as defined in Title I. The HSO provision was broad enough to accommodate solo practice physicians, organized in medical care foundations, and a minimum package of services that was not specified. Moreover, to ensure equal access and availability of services in a service area, Title III provided for establishment of a Health Maintenance Trust Fund to offer premium supplements (capitation grants) to people who could not afford to pay the membership premium of HMOs and HSOs.

The premium supplement was perhaps the most ingenious feature because it was a modest version of the payment mechanism to be employed by the Health Security Board to local health care organizations, under Kennedy's NHI program. Some critics would argue that the senator had backed a form of NHI into his HMO bill. Practically speaking, the size of the benefit package required by S.3327 would place the costs of an HMO membership well beyond the means of many people, who would, therefore, be entitled to a premium supplement to cover the difference between what they could afford and the costs of enrollment.

The supplement would enable HMOs to provide comprehensive benefits to all members of the community, regardless of income.

Another key provision of S.3327 was the establishment under Title IV of a Commission on Quality Health Care. The concept, the brainchild of Paul Ellwood, attempted to focus attention on "outcomes" of medical care, rather than on costs and medical procedures. Not surprisingly, it was the innovative Senate health subcommittee that embraced Ellwood's idea for a Health Outcomes Commission rather than the more conservative Senate Finance Committee.[41]

In summary, S.3327 limited the definition of HMOs to prepaid group practice plans; mandated a comprehensive package of required benefits; authorized expansive levels of federal support, including, in particular, a provision for premium supplements (capitation grants); defined specific quality assurance requirements and a Quality Assurance Commission to implement them; and provided sweeping authority for overriding restrictive state laws. Moreover, the bill introduced a new category of health care organization, an HSO (health service organization), which provided federal support to establish and operate solo practice medical foundations in rural areas, but not in urban areas; only "classic HMOs," prepaid group practice plans, would be encouraged in urban areas. Finally, the various provisions of the bill would cost a total of $5.1 billion over a five-year period of authorization.

S.3327 was an expansive, comprehensive, and ambitious proposal. Kennedy's motivations in constructing it were complex and cannot be ascribed solely to a desire to promote NHI through the back door.[42] His motives stemmed both from a belief in his appropriate role as a cutting edge for new and innovative health policies and also his unwillingness to

---

41. Ellwood had developed the concept primarily as a response to Senate Finance Committee criticism of HMOs as potential sources of "skimming" low-risk patients, while lowering health services quality, that is, "skimping." In his letter to Sen. Long in April 1972, urging reconsideration of various aspects of H.R.1's HMO provisions, Ellwood provided a succinct rationale for reliance on health outcomes monitoring and regulations, rather than paying inordinate attention to minute cost controls over medical procedures. See p. 103.
42. This argument was made by Sen. Peter Dominick (R-CO), principal committee critic of the bill, as cast by Kennedy. More precisely, Dominick called S.3327 a "promotional" bill, designed to transform the health care delivery system into a network of prepaid group practice plans. Kennedy's motivation appeared not to be establishment of an NHI program under the questionable jurisdiction of the Committee on Labor and Public Welfare, but to prepare the health care delivery system for the inevitability of NHI. To Kennedy's way of thinking, prepaid group practice plans were preferred, cost-effective mechanisms for delivering health care under the Health Security Program.

allow the first piece of legislation "ever put through the Congress that dealt with the matter of medical practice itself and the patterns of service delivery" to be vaguely conceived.[43]

Kennedy's preoccupation as chairman of the Senate health subcommittee was increasingly with the structure of health care delivery. Paradoxically, he and Caper shared a suspicion and skepticism of doctors and organized medicine comparable to that of Jay Constantine and the Senate Finance Committee. But, where Constantine and Long turned to the instrumentalities under their purview, regulations over Medicare and Medicaid reimbursements, that is, cost controls, Caper and Kennedy focused on their area of responsibility, the health care delivery system. In their own ways, both senators (and their staffs) tended to favor aggressive, activist federal postures — but within the range of options mandated by their congressional responsibilities. Ultimately, the prerogatives of power would dictate the shape of health system reform.

Kennedy was convinced that HMOs were proven, viable alternatives to fee-for-service medicine.[44] Since S.3327 was not an experimental or demonstration program, it was designed to ensure that HMOs would stimulate competition with the fee-for-service system by giving them a large push from the federal government. Thus, the twofold desire to ensure that HMOs would serve the public adequately and also have a fair chance to compete with fee-for-service medicine led inexorably to a large, expansive federal program. The public could be well served only if the benefit package were broad, groups of physicians were at financial risk, and elaborate quality assurance mechanisms were provided. These requirements, however, would demand substantial federal investments over a long period to expand the health system's resource capacities because no current HMOs could meet such ambitious service and quality assurance requirements. Similarly, the equally important objective of stimulating effective competition with the powerful fee-for-service system would require substantial subsidies (from the Health Maintenance trust fund) to make HMOs (as Kennedy conceived of them) financially competitive.[45]

---

43. Philip Caper, interview, June 1974.
44. Witness after witness, largely drawn from the labor movement and from advocates of the prepaid group practice movement, presented Kennedy with convincing evidence and arguments about the virtues of the HMO alternative. Only the AMA had negative comments, calling the concept unproven and, therefore, needing years of cautious, limited experimentation.
45. Because the premium supplements could only comprise 25 percent of an HMO's total receipts, however, it was questionable whether an HMO could compete with indem-

S.3327 proposed to convert the Nixon Administration's HMO proposal into a major new mechanism for federal intervention in health care systems. The Administration had argued that HMOs would lead to a lesser federal presence in health affairs. Kennedy, in contrast, sought to demonstrate that any serious challenge to prevailing health system behavior patterns could come about only through a quantum expansion of the federal role. Members of Assistant Secretary Lewis Butler's health planning staff in HEW had arrived at this same conclusion back in early 1970, when Ellwood first presented his HMO proposal. They used the spectre of a large federal role as a weapon against HMO. Now, two years later, Kennedy used the same arguments as a rationale for his huge HMO development program proposal.

Ellwood and HEW senior officials had prevailed and sold their concept to the White House largely on the promise that HMOs could offer a viable competitive alternative to fee-for-service medical care without requiring a massive federal commitment of resources. This assurance was predicated on two assumptions: first, that a modest federal (capital) investment program could stimulate the creation of a viable, competitive HMO alternative to fee-for-service medicine; second, that the HMO concept would generate a sufficient market presence to offer a viable alternative to the voluntary and indemnity health insurance plans.

Kennedy, Caper, and knowledgeable veterans of the prepaid group practice movement saw these promises as empty rhetoric. The prevailing system was a fee-for-service monopoly. How could a limited federal program possibly break this monopoly? Without significant federal resource commitments, the Administration's goal of 1,700 HMOs available to 90 percent of the population by 1977 was totally illusory.[46]

Furthermore, if HMOs were to become major competitive alternatives to indemnity insurance plans, a large federal development effort, on the order of Kennedy's proposals, would be required to create enough new HMOs to challenge the power of the established insurance plans. From his perspective, therefore, Kennedy was only obligating sufficient congressional monies to match the promise of Nixon's rhetoric.

---

nity plans and still provide a full complement of services. Because health care costs were inflating so rapidly, it might well be the case that no HMO could price its premium competitively, even after availing itself of the 25 percent supplement.

46. These goals were intemperately proposed in the Administration's White Paper, "Toward a Comprehensive Health Policy for the 1970s," published in the spring of 1971. Arguments urging caution had been unsuccessfully made in early 1970 by senior HEW health planners and Social Security Administration officials, who saw Paul Ellwood's proposal as much too grandiose for an Administration seeking to lower the federal health profile. Their arguments were prophetic. See chapter 2, pp. 35-38.

The Administration's reaction to Kennedy's proposals was quick and decidedly negative. Administration spokesmen saw S.3327 as totally unworkable. Kennedy's version of an HMO bore little resemblance to actual health plans successfully competing in the health care marketplace. The senator was trying to do more than extend current HMO prototypes to larger markets; he was trying to create new HMO prototypes of a kind that could never survive without substantial, permanent direct federal subsidies.

> This bill reflects a fundamentally different philosophy from the philosophy embodied in the Administration bill. It is not compatible with the Administration approach of seeking to develop economically self-sufficient organizations that can be viable in a competitive and pluralistic system. Indeed, it would finance a major reorganization of the health care delivery system on a heavily subsidized basis.[47]

Three HMO Bills: Differences To Be Reconciled

By the spring of 1972, a milestone in the legislative struggle had been reached with the completion of HMO assistance bills by the three principals in the unfolding debate. Each bill reflected the values, ideologies, and even prejudices of its author. H.R.5615, the Nixon Administration's contribution, articulated the flexible market incentive approach central to Nixon's health maintenance strategy. It was a loose bill, permitting a broad array of organizations to partake of federal assistance. In particular, H.R.5615 purposely did not spell out the service mixes to be provided by HMOs beyond such broad, generic categories as emergency care, inpatient hospital and physician care, ambulatory physician care, and outpatient preventive medical services. H.R.11728 offered tighter definitions and controls than H.R.5615, while S.3327 eclipsed both in its breadth and specificity.

On the key matter of the types of organizations that might qualify as an HMO, substantial differences existed among the three bills. Both the Roy and Kennedy bills referenced the term *medical group* in their definition of an HMO. Roy defined a medical group as a "partnership or other association of individuals"; Kennedy, however, substituted the phrase "not less than four persons" for the term *individuals.* This simple turn of phrase was to be the central focus of intense debate in Kennedy's health

---

47. Scott Fleming, "HMO Assistance-Kennedy Bill," memorandum from the Deputy Assistant Secretary for Health Policy to the Deputy Assistant Secretary for Health Legislation, HEW, Office of the Secretary, June 15, 1972.

subcommittee and, later, on the Senate floor. It effectively prohibited individual practice associations, usually organized as local medical society sponsored medical care foundations, from being considered as HMOs. It is absolutely certain that Caper intended such an exclusion.[48] Thus, solo practice physicians could not, in any way, qualify under this definition of an HMO.

Roy and his aide, Brian Biles, took a more benign position. Although clearly tilting toward the group practice model, they left the door open for individual practice associations, as previously noted. Both Roy and Kennedy indicated that professionals associated with an HMO would have to make the plan their principal professional activity and "engage in the coordinated practice of their profession as a group responsibility." But, since Roy had not precluded an "association of individuals" from qualifying, individual practice associations would meet the "coordinated practice as a group responsibility" requirement.[49] Kennedy and Caper, however, left no doubt that the reference to "coordination" and "group" could only apply to a closed panel, prepaid group practice plan.

Reimbursement arrangements were also subtly shaded in each bill to reflect the author's intent with regard to individual practices. Roy required all income to be pooled and distributed according to a prearranged plan or through an employment arrangement. Kennedy added the phrase "drawing account." Neither bill, according to these terms, precluded the basis of the reimbursement from being the dollar equivalent of what a physician would have received through a fee-for-service payment.

This language was sufficiently flexible to accommodate both Roy's "association of individuals" and Kennedy's secondary category of organization, "health service organizations (HSOs)." HSOs, to be established for rural and nonmetropolitan areas, did not have to meet the stringent service and organizational requirements of HMOs (that is,

---

48. Caper candidly told the Washington representative of the American Association of Foundations for Medical Care, James E. Bryan, who was trying to prevail upon him to accept a more flexible position, that "if we made foundation and individual practice plans equal to groups, we'd never get any closed panel groups." In other words, solo practice physicians, more numerous than group practice physicians, would overwhelm the HMO assistance program. Moreover, Caper believed that a major incentive for the recent rapid growth of foundation plans was the prospect of getting funds from the federal government. S.3327, therefore, was overtly favorable to closed panel, prepaid group practice plans.

49. Of course, such a plan would be less coordinated and much less responsible for patient care than a group. But, the degree of responsibility and "groupness" was left unstated in the Roy bill.

prepaid group practice plans) located in metropolitan areas. The logic behind the HSO concept was the reasonable presumption that greater scarcity of medical resources in nonmetropolitan areas would preclude an HSO from providing the full complement of comprehensive services required for HMOs.

Kennedy and Caper, therefore, proposed to relegate individual practice association medical foundation plans to rural areas. It was apparent that they viewed the geographical distances between providers, their limited number, and the scarcity of health care facilities associated with rural areas as the only compelling reasons to support organizations less structured than prepaid group practice plans.

H.R.5615, the Administration's bill, had the simplest organizational definition of an HMO: HMOs would provide "physicians' services" directly through physicians who were employees or partners of the HMO or "under arrangements with one or more groups of physicians organized on a group practice or individual practice basis." In short, there was little difference between Roy's and the Administration's definitions. The major departure was to be found in S.3327.

The participation of profit-making organizations was never an issue in S.3327. Caper and Kennedy astutely recognized the illusory nature of this distinction in the health sector. They knew their bill could not accomplish any sweeping changes unless substantial encouragement was offered for-profit health providers to participate in the program. After all, the source of the inflation in health care costs was not rooted in the Internal Revenue Code definitions of for-profit or not-for-profit corporate entities. In the present system, the most costly health service components, hospitals, were usually organized as not-for-profit entities. While the Senate Finance Committee could endlessly debate complex formulas for controlling "profits" or "rates of retention," Kennedy and Caper knew that the important factors were incentives, risks, the structure of health care organizations, and mechanisms for quality assurance. If the "right" organizational arrangements were established, the profit-making issue would be moot.

The Administration and Kennedy were in substantial agreement on the profit-making issue, essentially for the same reasons. The difference between them, however, was that Kennedy was not going out of his way to encourage the formation of profit-making entities. Therefore, S3327 provided only loan guarantees to profit-making entities. H.R.5615, however, provided for contracts to plan and develop profit-making HMOs, as well as loan guarantees to offset their initial operating losses. H.R.11728 reflected Roy's antipathy for profit-making health care organizations and covered only nonprofit and public organizations.

The Senate and House bills provided for fixed, uniform payments for all members on the basis of "community rating."[50] But the House version exempted beneficiaries under Medicare and Medicaid, or others authorized by the Secretary. The Senate exempted no population segments, while the Administration bill had no provision at all regarding population groups.

All three bills provided for an annual open enrollment period.[51] But the Roy and Administration bills exempted HMOs from this provision with regard to Medicare enrollment and as waived by the Secretary. Open enrollment in the Kennedy bill was unconditional.

The Administration made no specific provision for consumer participation. The Roy bill called for consumers to play a "meaningful role in the making of policy" and to have access to meaningful grievance procedures. Kennedy added a requirement that there be "equitable representation" from medically underserved areas. Although not specifically requiring consumer membership on an HMO's board of directors, priority funding would nevertheless be given to HMOs that made such provision.

The Administration bill did not include a provision to override restrictive state legislation that prohibited the organization and incorporation of HMOs.[52] Their position reflected the Republican preference for working through state and local instrumentalities, whenever possible. The Administration would, therefore, encourage states to remove such restrictions and would provide them with technical assistance to rewrite their medical practice incorporation laws. This approach was designed so as not to upset states' rights-oriented conservatives of either party.[53]

---

50. Community rating is an insurance industry term meaning that the actuarial risks (of illness) in a community will be averaged, so that high-risk groups and low-risk groups will each receive the same risk rating and, therefore, the same premium. Experience rating, in contrast, establishes specific classes of actuarial risk for different population groups (or even for individual employed groups) and establishes differential premiums for each group.
51. Open enrollment is a concept designed to guard against adverse selection, or "skimming," of low-risk groups, to the disadvantage of high-risk groups. It seeks to complement a community rating system, by ensuring that either an HMO or conventional health insurance plan cannot turn away less desirable subscribers, even though, because of community rating, they will pay the same fixed premium as more desirable (lower risk) enrollees.
52. By 1970, 22 states had incorporated, in one form or another, restrictive legislation, primarily at the urging of state and county medical societies. The effect of such laws was to give solo practice, fee-for-service providers a professional monopoly.
53. The AMA was able to capitalize on the state override provision issue, later in 1972 and 1973, particularly with Republican members of the House health subcommittee.

Both the House and Senate bills, however, contained override provisions. There was one subtle difference between the two approaches. S.3327 simply invalidated the restrictive statutes, allowing the organization to proceed under state laws of incorporation or licensure. Roy would authorize the Secretary of HEW to issue a certificate of incorporation directly to the prospective HMO, thereby nullifying the effects of the restrictive state law. This offered the organization federally mandated incorporation, possibly calling into question state laws of incorporation and medical licensure procedures.[54]

A significant omission from all bills was any reference to "mandatory, dual, or multiple choice." Ellwood had advocated such a provision in his earliest days working with the Administration. Later in 1972, during committee markups of the bills, the dual choice issue was squarely confronted.[55]

On the question of federal support, the Senate proposal was an omnibus bill, promising comprehensive federal intervention into the health care delivery system. A five-year authorization of $5.1 billion was suggested. Both the House and Administration bills were much more modest ventures. The big issue raised by these contrasting authorizations was the extent to which the federal government should intervene in the health care delivery system. Would the Kennedy approach be accepted, that is, a full-scale, virtually permanent federal program? Or would Congress settle for a more limited venture? A subsidiary issue was the question of whether HMOs were now considered proven entities. If they were, then a full-scale federal commitment might be justified. But if they required more years of research and development, a more modest

---

54. Detailed analytical work on ways to implement the override of restrictive state laws was undertaken by American Rehabilitation Foundation staff in 1971. ARF testimony before both House and Senate health subcommittees urged that explicit language be included in subsequent markups. For a detailed review, see: Rick J. Carlson. "State/Federal Relationships." *Proceedings: Lawyers Conference on Health Maintenance Organizations.* Aug. 20-21, 1971, pp. 62-76.

55. "Mandatory dual choice" is a technique designed to offer HMOs equal access to the marketplace, by requiring employers to offer their employees an HMO option as part of their health insurance benefit plans. This principle engendered little controversy until specific language found its way into subsequent (markup) bills. The provision remained in the House version and was included, then subsequently deleted, from S.3327. Organized labor had difficulty accepting a potential intrusion into the collective bargaining process. The final HMO development bill, passed by Congress, did include a mandatory dual-choice provision. Its implementation almost immediately became the subject of dispute between HEW, organized labor, the Department of Labor, and the National Labor Relations Board. Labor's fears that HEW would misuse the new authority proved to be entirely justified by ensuing events. See chapter 7, pp. 168-169, for a full account of this controversy.

demonstration effort would be more appropriate. The semantic meaning of words such as *full effort, demonstration,* and *experimental program* became subjects of extended debate.

H.R.5615 and H.R.11728 provided, in general terms, that arrangements must be made to ensure quality. The Roy bill, however, specified that quality assurance procedures must stress medical care processes and "outcomes." The Administration bill only suggested that health services be received "promptly" and "appropriately."

Once again, the big departure was found in S.3327. Title IV would establish a Commission on Quality Health Care Assurance, an independent federal regulatory agency, with detailed and specific mandates to establish standards and prescribe quality control systems for HMOs, HSOs, and other providers. This commission would also be empowered to undertake data development studies, absorbing the National Center for Health Statistics, and it would be responsible for a medical malpractice insurance fund.

Because S.3327 spelled out an expensive benefit package and required at least 30 percent enrollment from medically underserved areas, "capitation grants" were to be available to HMOs to offset the gap between per capita premium costs and what enrollees could be "expected to pay." Poor people, in short, were not to be deprived of opportunities for enrollment. However, no more than 25 percent of total HMO premium receipts could come from capitation grants. To pay these premiums, the government would establish a Health Maintenance trust fund, to be financed largely by crediting 5 percent of taxes from alcoholic beverages, cigarettes, and other tobacco products.[56]

* * *

In summary, the three HMO assistance bills under consideration during 1972 were substantially different in important ways. Their differences reflected not just the political and professional tastes of Roy, Kennedy, Biles, and Caper, although Biles and Caper had a virtual carte blanche in

---

56. The tax features of the trust fund were clever. By using alcohol and cigarette taxes as subsidies for the health care of low-income people, Kennedy and Caper were, in effect, forcing both drinkers and smokers to pay for a portion of the health care of the nation. The health-threatening vices of some would support the health care of others. However, the provision smacked of "back-door" national health insurance to critics of S.3327. Moreover, the tax provisions would require a discharge from the Senate Finance Committee, which would have to agree to allow the establishment of the new trust fund and its permanent funding through the federal tax system.

constructing their respective HMO assistance bills. The contrasts reflected, to a great extent, the perspectives and philosophies of the interests that would be affected by the outcome of the legislative struggle. As specific issues and options came into focus during the long months of HMO bill writing and markup, these interests began to focus on health maintenance. The year 1973 would be pivotal as both the pace of debate and its intensity quickened with the growing realization of the major health interest groups that the passage of HMO enabling legislation was a very real possibility.

CHAPTER 6

The Legislative Struggle: Part II

Interest groups play a prominent role in America's pluralistic political system. How these groups articulate their policies and how they seek to influence the institutions of public authority have been major topics in the literature of political science. Interest groups exercise varying degrees of influence, depending upon the structure of particular sectors of the political economy and the parochial nature of issues that reach the public agenda.

The health sector has been characterized as a mixed public-private system, with most resources and services produced and distributed by private organizations and professionals organized in guildlike professional societies. Public sector activities focus on regulation, licensure, and financial support of these private sector professions and organizations. Private health interest groups are important in the health sector because effective governmental performance depends on the accuracy and timeliness of public authorities' knowledge about resource producers, service providers, and rapidly evolving health care technologies. Such information is essential if public authorities hope to promulgate appropriate health-related laws and regulations.[1]

1. Organized interests actively influence and shape governmental roles in the political economy. In the health sector, the interests of medical providers, allied health professionals, hospitals, and medical center-teaching research complexes have

Health interest groups use their favored access to federal, state, and local public officials to lobby for favorable treatment for their constituents. New policies and programs have often been originated by these organizations. Landmark legislation to support hospital construction (the Hill-Burton Program) resulted directly from the efforts of the American Hospital Association. Similarly, the dramatic growth of federal support for biomedical research into causes and cures of the dread diseases has been, in large part, a response to the aggressive lobbying of health scientists and civic-minded philanthropists, who form the influential medical research lobby.[2]

In recent years, as the scope of the federal government's health activities has sharply increased — particularly in financing medical services and research — the voices of consumer representatives, labor federations, taxpayer organizations, and a growing band of cost-conscious governmental and private analysts have begun to be heard, calling for greater prudence in the allocation of increasingly scarce health dollars. The Health Maintenance Plan was a response to this call for greater cost-effectiveness in the field of medical care. The strategy was the product of the newer, rather than of the older, established health interests. It emerged without benefit of guidance from the established health interest groups that had shaped the health policies of earlier periods. These policies, in fact, were being vigorously challenged by the advocates of HMO: the energetic efforts of the American Rehabilitation Foundation (ARF), working closely with its professional counterparts at HEW; the Group Health Association of America (GHAA); and the American Association of Foundations for Medical Care (AAFMC). HMO strategy development in 1970 and 1971 was notable because of its insulation from most of the traditional, established health interest groups and for the ascendancy of these newer groups.

Advocates and Opponents

Paul Ellwood had greatly underestimated the protracted nature of the legislative struggle over HMOs. As 1971 dragged on with no early

---

dominated the politics of health. In recent years, consumers of health have become more effective in challenging the virtual monopoly of provider and producer access to the nation's health policy. For an excellent description of interest group politics in the health sector, see: Alford, Robert A. *Health Care Politics: Ideological and Interest Group Barriers to Reform.* Chicago: University of Chicago Press, 1975.

2. For an authoritative account of the role of the medical research lobby, see: Stephen P. Strickland, *Politics, Science, and Dread Disease.* Cambridge, MA: Harvard, 1972.

prospect of action on the HMO assistance bills, it became clear that the heavily Democratic 92nd Congress was not about to rubberstamp any legislative offering, however meritorious, of a Republican President highly disliked by so many. Thus, when a routine request for ARF comments came from Brian Biles as he was drafting the House bill, it represented a welcome opportunity for ARF to broaden its HMO advocacy into the legislature.

Two of ARF's professional staff, Patrick O'Donoghue, M.D., and Rick Carlson, a lawyer, took the lead in responding to the congressional overture. Biles came to have a very high regard for O'Donoghue and Carlson, considering them

> . . . the best lobbyists I've seen since I've been in Washington. They would hit town and would start at OMB and then go to HEW and then come on the Democratic side and then on the Republican side and they would just make the rounds. And they were very, very discreet. . . .[3]

It was also useful to have some people around who could freely communicate across party lines, between Senate and House health subcommittees and legislative and executive branches. O'Donoghue observed:

> We to some extent played the role of intermediary . . . deliberately. . . . We didn't do anything we weren't told to do, but Administration people [would] say, why don't you call up the Kennedy subcommittee and try that idea out on them? . . .[4]

Trustworthy communicators are vital to the political process; and ARF's identification as the HMO think tank gave it an aura of nonpartisanship not possessed by other groups that represented particular clienteles. ARF's partisanship was to the HMO concept itself.

Advising the staff of congressional health subcommittees, however, called for a new strategy, one that recognized their predisposition to draw highly specific laws and to mandate detailed regulations. The HMO "market reform" model that Ellwood had recommended to a Republican Administration did not receive a very positive response from Democratic subcommittees comfortable only with a large federal presence and the regulations to back that presence up. Tactically, O'Donoghue and Carlson displayed considerable flexibility and willingness to work within guidelines they were not necessarily in agreement with. "We were willing

---

3. Brian Biles, interview, June 1974.
4. Patrick O'Donoghue, M.D., interview, Oct. 1974.

to say, it was best to do A, but given that you want to do either B or C, then choose B," they said.[5]

A long-range strategy, however, had to help shape options, not merely guide choices among a limited range of less desirable alternatives. Two aspects of a congressional strategy began to take shape late in 1971: one was a plan to focus congressional enthusiasm for regulations into channels constructive to HMO development; a second was to develop unique ARF positions on each of the critical elements in the legislative struggle and to try to nudge the health subcommittees in those directions. "Quality assurance" provided an opportunity to design a regulatory approach supportive of HMOs. Beyond that key element of HMO legislation, other issues called for ARF's attention, issues such as greater flexibility of organizational requirements for HMOs, a limited benefit package, equalization of market opportunities through mandatory dual choice, and preemption of restrictive state laws.

Critics of prepaid group practice often suggested that the services delivered by such plans were of a poorer quality than services provided under fee-for-service practice. ARF believed that the best way to counter such claims would be to ensure high-quality services by installing a comprehensive quality assurance mechanism in HMOs. The focus would be on health outcomes and the HMO quality assurance system would be regulated by a Health Outcomes Commission. ARF research produced the core of a comprehensive quality assurance program for HMOs. The program called for the establishment of a Health Outcomes Commission to monitor HMOs and other providers were to be encouraged to come under the commission's jurisdiction, as well. Initially, the program was presented to HEW, which balked at its elaborate regulatory approach and its reliance on outcome measures. "Then we said, in effect, to the Administration, that we really believed in the program and should present our findings objectively to anyone that is interested."[6]

In January 1972, preliminary conclusions were drawn together into a draft monograph as the principal discussion document for an ARF-sponsored conference on quality assurance in New Orleans.[7] Forty-seven people, representing a wide variety of health system expertise, assembled to hear the ARF proposals and to critique them. They were generally critical of the quality assurance program. But their exposure to the ideas

---

5. *Ibid.*
6. *Ibid.*
7. Paul M. Ellwood Jr., M.D., and others. *Assuring the Quality of Health Care.* Minneapolis, MN: InterStudy, 1973, pp. 1-2.

was a significant milestone for the HMO policy process: among the 47 attendees was Kennedy's aide, Philip Caper, who picked up the Health Outcomes Commission idea and incorporated it as Title IV of S.3327, the Senate HMO development bill.

*   *   *

The Group Health Association of America (GHAA) was also a key proponent of the HMO concept. It was hardly surprising that congressional health subcommittee staffs sought GHAA guidance on their evolving legislation. As the premier membership organization for the nation's prototype HMOs, prepaid group practice plans, GHAA staff was regularly consulted during the bill-writing process and played a pivotal role as a counterbalance to AMA efforts to kill the HMO initiative. For very different reasons from those of the AMA, however, GHAA began to have serious doubts about the shape of HMO legislation during the spring and summer of 1972. While never wavering in its basic support of an HMO assistance bill, GHAA wished to shape a bill that its membership could live with. The basis for an hospitable relationship between government and established prepaid group practice plans could be found in Roy's bill, H.R.11728, with certain amendments deriving from the Administration's bill. In general, GHAA believed that attempts to force greater responsibilities on HMOs by requiring large benefit packages, mandatory coverage of too many poor people, and excessively onerous reporting requirements and quality controls would cause difficulties for current or newly established plans.

GHAA's goal, therefore, was to secure passage of a practical, workable HMO bill. From this perspective, it had great difficulty with the comprehensive nature of S.3327. It was unlikely that currently operating prepaid group practice plans, or any likely to be formed in the foreseeable future, could hope to meet its stringent requirements. Most of GHAA's attention, therefore, was focused on the House Commerce health subcommittee. A central concern was the size of the benefit package: H.R.11728 mandated too many services to be covered by a fixed-price premium; the appropriate package would be the four minimum services suggested in the Administration's bill, H.R.5615, but with the addition of diagnostic laboratory and diagnostic and therapeutic radiological services. The costs of providing the full range of services mandated under H.R.11728 would be too great to permit an HMO to compete in the health marketplace. Ernest W. Saward, M.D., chairman of GHAA's board of directors, stated his organization's belief that "if comprehensive services are spread to very broad limits, it prices the package out of the insurance market. . . . Therefore, . . . comprehensiveness should not be a starting requirement.[8]

From the outset, GHAA saw federal entry into the HMO field as a mixed blessing. On the one hand, only with federal aid could the prepaid group practice type of HMOs ever hope to expand rapidly. Progress over the past 40 years, while definite, had nonetheless been slow. Federal assistance could sharply increase the pace of development. There was a danger, however, that the congressional tendency to overpromise the benefits of reform programs and to misread the capacity or willingness of entrenched health system interests to respond to federal initiatives could place HMOs at a competitive disadvantage with indemnity insurance plans and fee-for-service medicine. Saward, in his testimony, had caught the nuance correctly by emphasizing the words *aid* and *assist*. *Aid* and *assist* what? Surely not some abstract utopian system of health care but "real world" HMO prototypes that could be replicated across the nation.

S.3327 was a developmental and promotional bill seeking to create new health care delivery systems not currently existing anywhere in the nation. GHAA took particular exception to the mandatory provision of 12 separate health services and urged the Kennedy subcommittee on health to reduce drastically these requirements.

A second GHAA concern was with the rapid and coincidental growth of the medical foundation movement. As related in chapter 2, medical care foundations have a relatively recent history, tracing their origin to the formation of the San Joaquin Medical Foundation in 1954. Their growth, in the intervening years, had been slow, accelerating somewhat in the late 1960s and early 1970s. GHAA believed that this growth was an overt response to the challenge of (prepaid group practice) HMOs. This was true, in part. As the tempo of HMO policy development increased, so, too, did the efforts of foundation plans. Their objective was to make certain that any federal program of HMO assistance would define the HMO concept broadly enough to include them. Foundation plans, however, had predated by some years, in origin, the formal commitment of the federal government to HMO development in 1971. Their formation was a response to other forces in the evolution of health care systems — not just to the challenge of group practice-type HMOs. Foundation

---

8. Ernest W. Saward, M.D., Testimony on HMO Enabling Legislation, Hearings on Health Maintenance Organizations, Part I, before the Subcommittee on Health and the Environment, U.S. House of Representatives, Apr. 1972, Serial No. 92-88, p. 184.

plans also responded to the challenge to set up peer review standards and guidance, under medical society auspices, for private practitioners. The plans offered a method for internal self-policing to improve the quality of office-based general medical practice.

Because foundation plans represented more modest rearrangements of medical care practice than group practice plans, they were tacitly accepted by the AMA as a somewhat preferred option to the more radical changes that would accompany prepaid group practice. However, the AMA never aggressively supported or promoted the formation of foundation medical plans.[9]

Neither was GHAA opposed to medical care foundations receiving attention under HMO assistance legislation. Rather, GHAA believed that Congress should recognize the differences between these two types of HMOs and fund each appropriately. This would mean restricting foundation plans' access to facilities construction funds (inasmuch as services were normally provided out of physicians' offices, not out of new facilities). Neither should they have their initial operating costs offset "because subscribers to such programs are simply an addition to or substitute for those already making fee-for-service payments to practitioners."[10]

GHAA also took exception to the detailed reporting requirements of H.R.11728 and S.3327, the open enrollment requirement, and the mandatory enrollment of 30 percent from medically underserved areas proposed in S.3327. Each of these provisions, as written, put greater burdens on HMOs than were placed upon indemnity health insurance plans. The paradox seemed clear enough: the health insurance industry, unencumbered with public responsibilities, would continue to be free to pursue subscribers, governed only by rather benign rules pertaining to insurance industry practices established by the several states. HMOs, charged with heavy public responsibilities and special conditions upon their receipt of federal assistance, would have to undertake missions that would make it impossible for them to compete with the indemnity insurers. Caper, the author of S.3327, maintained that, after all, no one was coercing anyone else to participate in the proposed federal program.[11] This argument, however, totally ignored the practical realities of the health care marketplace: if health providers found no incentives in a federal program, why would they try to participate? Or, conversely, could

---

9. Memorandum on issues on HMO legislation, GHAA, 1972.
10. *Ibid.*
11. Philip Caper, interview, June 1974.

HMOs afford *not* to participate, knowing that some of their competitors were likely to seek and receive federal aid? GHAA believed that the Kennedy bill was unrealistic, however well-intentioned its motives:

> . . . we had several problems with the Kennedy bill. Our specific objections were directed toward the size of the benefit package and the Commission on Quality Care. In addition, there was general objection to the large financial commitment authorized by the Kennedy legislation.[12]

There was little hope that Kennedy would moderate his position. S.3327 would pass, essentially as Kennedy had proposed it, a testimonial to his dominance of health care legislation in the Senate. But the prospects for ultimate passage of an HMO program in the 92nd Congress were appreciably diminished by the passage of S.3327. There was little enthusiasm on the part of House Commerce health subcommittee members to go into a conference with the Senate and to try to reconcile two bills so vastly different in scope and purpose. For, while Kennedy was rapidly maneuvering S.3327 through subcommittee hearings and full Labor and Public Welfare Committee clearance, the House health subcommittee was undertaking a painstaking, section-by-section markup of H.R.11728. The willingness of Rogers and his subcommittee to consider the HMO bill so carefully provided a favorable environment for GHAA to secure greater flexibility in the ultimate House bill. At the same time, the delay in House consideration meant that the Senate could commit itself to an omnibus bill, unrestrained by a more moderate House yardstick.

* * *

The American Association of Foundations for Medical Care (AAFMC) represents the interests of the other major HMO prototype: individual practice associations (IPAs), or foundations for medical care (FMCs). The first foundation plan was established in 1954, in the rural San Joaquin County of California, in direct response to the growing presence of the Kaiser-Permanente Health Care Program, the nation's largest and most successful prepaid group practice plan. The solo practice physicians of the county viewed the success of Kaiser and its potential expansion into their valley with alarm and established the San Joa-

---

12. James Doherty, "HMO Legislation," memorandum to the field staff, GHAA, Oct. 31, 1972.

quin County Foundation for Medical Care, a legal subdivision of the county medical society.

The San Joaquin FMC kept Kaiser out of the San Joaquin Valley and proved that fixed-sum prepayment could be harmonized with solo practice fee-for-service medical practice, yielding significant improvements in cost efficiency and medical care quality. The FMC movement spread throughout California, engaging the Kaiser plans in vigorous competition for enrollment, in many locales.

The California-based FMCs organized themselves into a self-help association called the United Foundations for Medical Care, in the late 1950s. By the late 1960s, with the spread of the foundation approach to 11 other states and plans for foundations in 25 more, the originators of the California programs decided to establish a national association: the result was the incorporation of AAFMC, in January 1971. The services of an experienced Washington representative were retained on a part-time basis, and the assignment fell to James E. Bryan, who had previously served in a similar capacity for the Blue Shield Plans. Bryan's initial assignment was to establish a listening post for AAFMC, particularly with regard to congressional consideration of two health care reforms that would most affect the fortunes of FMCs: Professional Standards Review Organizations (PSROs) and HMOs.

Early contacts with Roy and his staff indicated that FMCs would receive favorable consideration in the House version of HMO legislation. The situation in the Senate was just the opposite: by late 1971, the shape of Kennedy's approach was coming into focus. It was highly unfavorable to FMCs. Much of the AAFMC focus during 1972 and 1973, therefore, centered on trying to convert an unfavorable climate of opinion in the Senate health subcommittee to one favorable to FMCs.

The evolving position of Kennedy, as articulated by Caper, was fivefold: first, FMCs were alleged to be organized medicine's reaction to the challenge of prepaid group practice (PPGP); second, because FMCs utilized existing community health facilities and resources, they ought not to have access to the same front-end federal investments that were required by PPGPs; third, fee-for-service medicine was flourishing and, therefore, the federal government should not promote it at the expense of the development of new PPGPs; fourth, because PPGP is the classic HMO prototype, FMCs could not be included in the basic HMO definitions; and fifth, the only proper field for FMCs was in rural areas where the conditions to establish closed-panel PPGPs did not exist.

AAFMC worked hard to dispel these objections, which were, on the whole, distortions of the history and experience of FMCs. Leaders of AAFMC had never denied that FMCs were spawned out of the challenges of PPGP encroachment on fee-for-service practice. Nevertheless, it could not be claimed that PPGPs were the only viable response to the crisis in health care costs and quality. At every opportunity, AAFMC emphasized the positive impact of FMCs on the same problems also being addressed by PPGPs; in foundation plan communities, hospital admission rates and average lengths of stay had been substantially reduced; there were also significant expansions in the range of services available because of the foundations' insistence on comprehensive benefit packages.[13]

Moreover, it was highly misleading to lump FMCs in with "organized medicine," the code words for the AMA. Public statements by AMA officials to the contrary notwithstanding, the AMA was no partisan of FMCs or of the AAFMC.[14] In the last analysis, orthodox AMA opinion saw FMCs as slightly less dangerous threats to fee-for-service medicine than PPGPs.[15] AAFMC officials took issue with AMA's position that there should be no federal legislative assistance for HMOs. Their Washington representative considered this AMA stance "feeble" and "an abdication of leadership."[16]

The FMCs were determined to qualify as HMOs, in order to benefit from the marketing opportunities and reimbursement provisions of an HMO assistance law. Without the ability to qualify, the growth of FMCs nationally would be inhibited and an unfair advantage given to the rival PPGPs. Thus, acceptance as an HMO was required as much for its symbolic significance as for any benefits to be gained from federal funding.

Caper maintained, throughout the spring of 1972, that no subsidies should go to FMCs. "Fee-for-service is here and flourishing — why should the government spend any more money to encourage it?"[17] AAFMC conceded that FMCs would not require capital funds for facilities construction as would PPGPs. Caper may well have been correct in his fear that, if given official parity with PPGPs, even in the

---

13. James E. Bryan, interview, Jan. 1978.
14. *Ibid.*
15. AMA Executive Vice-President Ernest B. Howard, M.D., believed that fee-for-service might not be able to survive under an FMC's prepaid arrangement. Quoted in "And Never the Twain Shall Meet," *Medical World News,* Dec. 3, 1971.
16. James E. Bryan, letter to the Executive Director of the AAFMC, Nov. 19, 1971.
17. Philip Caper, quoted by James E. Bryan in memorandum to the President and Executive Director of the AAFMC, May 19, 1972.

federal definition of an HMO, FMCs would outstrip their organizational counterparts as preferred developmental alternatives. To AAFMC's representatives, however, this was a grudging admission of both the attractiveness of the FMC option to the medical community and of its utility as an innovation in health services organization.

Finally, the decision to relegate FMCs to the rural hinterlands could be justified only if the federal government were arrogating to itself the final say as to preferred types of medical practices to be established in cities and rural areas. Certainly, the rapid expansion of the FMC concept into heavily populated states and localities offered strong evidence that foundation plans were viable in urban areas as well as in rural areas.

The AAFMC undertook an intensive lobbying effort to modify S.3327 so that FMCs would be treated equally with PPGPs. Key foundation presidents from around the nation wrote to members of the Senate Labor and Public Welfare Committee, urging that they give equal opportunity to FMCs and PPGPs.

> To restrict foundations to operating in rural areas as Health Service Organizations (as this bill presently would do) is unrealistic, impracticable, and would preclude competition for free choice of plan for the patient.[18]

Sen. Peter Dominick (R-CO), a senior member of the health subcommittee, had been educated to the FMC concept through the efforts of the Colorado State FMC and AAFMC's Washington representative. Dominick and his aide, Charles Woodruff, tried to modify S.3327 in subcommittee, but were only partially successful: the marked-up version, reported out by the full Labor and Public Welfare Committee on June 21, 1972, added a Section B to Title I, creating a new category, called "Supplemental HMOs," which would accommodate the FMC. However, Section 1108 allowed them to be funded only after all Section A HMOs, that is, PPGPs, had been funded, or after the Secretary certified that no more PPGPs were available for funding. "The effect of the word 'supplemental' is to rate the individual practice foundation pattern of medical service as secondary to closed panel group practice — the tail wagging the dog."[19] Dominick vigorously protested the discriminatory provisions of S.3327, and filed individual (dissenting) views with the committee report. He promised to continue the fight on the Senate floor with a series of

18. James E. Bryan, memorandum to AAFMC members, June 6, 1972.
19. James E. Bryan, Subject: HMO Legislation, memorandum to the Executive Director of the AAFMC, June 30, 1972.

amendments designed to liberalize the definition of an HMO to include the FMC, and to reduce the scale of the bill to more manageable proportions.

Kennedy, meanwhile, was angered by AAFMC's vigorous efforts on behalf of FMCs as well as by the AMA's attempt to delay consideration of S.3327. In a statement to his senate colleagues, urging prompt consideration of S.3327, Kennedy

> assumed, or at least tried to get others to conclude, that AAFMC was in total collusion with AMA in its efforts to kill the HMO bill. Actually, his people who drew this story knew better than that, but it didn't serve his purpose to draw any of these fine distinctions.[20]

* * *

The Washington staff of AMA had long accepted the inevitability of a permanent federal presence in the health sector. It knew that the watershed had been passed in 1965, when, after its most vigorous lobbying effort in recent history, the AMA could not block passage of the Medicare program. With such a large foot in the door, it was inevitable that the federal government would seek to protect its ever growing investments with further statutory and regulatory interventions in health and medical affairs.[21] Significant elements of the AMA leadership, however, remained totally unreconciled to a permanent role for the federal government in health care delivery matters. Most elected officials of the organization were adamant in their opposition to any federal support of HMOs. A degree of ambivalence, therefore, is discernible in the AMA's behavior with regard to HMO policy. The professional lobbyists in

---

20. James E. Bryan, letter to the executive director of the AAFMC, Sept. 1, 1972.
21. The "foot in the door" hypothesis is consistent with the widely accepted theory of American politics known as "incrementalism." According to this concept, change and innovation in American politics come about through small, stepwise increments to established policies. Designers of the Medicare legislative strategy have acknowledged their acceptance of the incremental approach. I. S. Falk, Wilbur Cohen, Nelson Cruikshank, and others had been seeking an NHI program unsuccessfully since the 1930s, when they were unable to dissuade President Roosevelt from dropping the proposal, under intense AMA pressure, from his original Social Security package. Periodic failures in the 1940s led these strategists to a more limited focus on the poor and the elderly. In 1965, the last critical compromise was made: no "cap" would be put on the new federal payment programs; costs and fees would be reimbursed without imposing restraints on medicine's private pricing structure. The Medicare strategists knew, however, that once the law was put on the books, the federal government would have to develop further policies to protect their growing investment.

Washington believed AMA's appropriate role was to seek access to federal health policymakers and try to limit or shape any given intrusion. However, the AMA leadership, in Chicago, wanted the HMO policy stopped cold.

In 1971, AMA staff had reacted with indifference to Rep. William Roy's efforts to draft his own HMO bill. Although the staff member who concentrated on the Democratic membership, Howard Lee Cook, had warned that Rep. Paul Rogers, health subcommittee chairman, had promised to cosponsor Roy's bill when it was ready for introduction, only after this prediction came true and hearings were scheduled for the spring of 1972 did the AMA take the HMO initiative seriously.[22] If Rogers wanted HMOs, then he would probably get them.

AMA strategy for dealing with HMOs finally began to move in a coherent direction early in 1972. The organization particularly opposed federal subsidization of formation of prepaid group practice plans as a competitive alternative to fee-for-service medical practice. Ostensibly, the opposition was to federal *subsidization* of HMOs, not to HMOs *per se.* If HMOs could survive on their own in the free market, then they deserved a place on the medical care landscape. It would be improper, however, for the federal government to tilt such a market test unfairly toward HMOs.[23]

Publicly, AMA had no objections to limited federal experimentation with HMOs, on a magnitude not significantly larger than the 110 projects supported by HEW under extant authorities, through early 1972. Any larger commitment would be an unwarranted intrusion. To reinforce this position, AMA lobbyists pointed out to Rogers that HEW had made substantial commitments to HMOs without congressional authorization at a time when Congress was considering its own program. As we have seen, Rogers joined Kennedy in urging HEW Secretary Elliot Richardson to end such experimentation until Congress could present the executive branch with a unique HMO mandate. Richardson reluctantly acceded to their wishes.

A two-tiered AMA strategy toward HMO emerged: public support for the HMO concept (while taking every opportunity to point out faults) and intensive private lobbying efforts to kill pending federal HMO legislation. This strategy moved forward in 1972 on a number of fronts.

---

22. Howard Lee Cook, interview, Aug. 1974.
23. Obviously, the counterargument that the entire extant health care market was unfairly monopolized by fee-for-service solo practitioners was unsympathetically received.

Initial efforts involved presentations by AMA board members before Senate and House hearings. In these forums, the basic public posture was articulated: HMOs were important parts of a pluralistic health care system but were unproven in the ways suggested by their advocates. Therefore, the federal government should proceed with considerable caution and not tie public resources to open-ended commitments for HMOs. Accompanying this public position was an "HMO Fact Sheet" and a "Medical Backgrounder," designed specifically to cast doubt on some of the more ambitious claims about HMOs. These documents focused on problems HMOs have had, such as underutilization, quality assurance, insolvency, and the costs to start and maintain them. The idea was to focus congressional attention on the potential weaknesses of HMOs, to counteract the propaganda of HMO advocates such as Ellwood, and to put them on the defensive. "The best defense is a good offense. I'd rather have the HMO advocates . . . on the defensive."[24]

A particularly ingenious argument was to point out the inconsistency in the HMO advocates' position on whether or not the HMO was a proven concept. Some argued that funds were needed to experiment with different HMO models. Other advocates, in different forums, maintained that HMOs had proven their viability, warranting a large federal commitment. If the HMO was a proven concept in the health care marketplace, reasoned the AMA, then why would HMOs require substantial investments from the federal government? Their "proven" track record ought to be sufficient to gain them wide acceptance. However, if HMOs were unproven, wouldn't a large federal commitment be capricious? Finally, while there was a precedent for federal demonstrations of alternative models of health care delivery, why should HMOs warrant any greater attention than any other experimental programs?

The AMA critiques then focused on HEW's own growth projections from their 1971 white paper, "Toward a Comprehensive Health Policy for the 1970s," and indicated to congressmen that passage of an HMO development bill, regardless of proposed authorization levels, would, in fact, cost much more than HEW's estimates. The white paper projected 1,700 HMOs begun by 1977.[25] The AMA used a base amount of $7.6 million as a start-up cost figure (the cost to the United Auto Workers of

24. Wayne Bradley, interview, Sept. 1974.

25. The projection of future HMO operations became a rather slippery numbers game. By late 1972, in fact, HEW had revised its estimates down to 1,210 HMOs by 1980. Of course, these estimates proved to be outrageously overstated. By 1978, there were only 203 prepaid health plans.

establishing its Detroit-based HMO during the 1950s). If the Detroit experience was indicative of the costs of other HMO starts, then an HMO development program of the magnitude suggested by HEW planners would cost $13 billion.[26]

These arguments were presented principally to minority (Republican) members of the House Commerce health subcommittee. Because the Republican minority had no staff until 1973, they depended on AMA information sources to help form their opinions on complex pieces of legislation, such as HMOs. In 1972, AMA strategists filled this informational gap well for the conservative congressmen.

The Senate health subcommittee was almost completely indifferent to AMA lobbying. The Democrats were liberals and oriented toward the labor movement. The ranking Republican was the liberal Javits. Schweiker, another ranking Republican, then had one of the most liberal voting records in the Senate. Only Dominick could be counted on to take an active and sustained conservative position in health matters. And his support of AMA positions was highly conditional.[27]

Kennedy's proposal was frightening in its scope and sweep, threatening to replace the health care delivery system with something alien and hostile to the fee-for-service brand of medicine. S.3327 also presented the real spectre of at least partially finding its way into statute, if it ever got into conference committee with the far more modest House version. Health legislation, having once reached the floor of either house of Congress, would have a good chance of being enacted. HMO legislation had to be stopped cold in the House Commerce Committee, if it was to be stopped at all. "Our strategy was that there would be no HMO bill in the 92nd Congress . . . because the Senate bill was so bad, anything that came out of conference we were afraid of."[28] S.3327, therefore, was the principal reason for the hardening position of the AMA toward HMOs as 1972 progressed. Kennedy's "opening to the left" really frightened the

26. The AMA's use of the $7.6 million figure, while high, was in the ballpark. HEW estimates put the initial development and start-up costs of HMOs around $3-5 million. In other words, both advocates and opponents were in substantial agreement that matching HEW's rhetoric with appropriations would commit public funds far in excess of even the lavishly funded Kennedy proposal. HEW, of course, argued that its use of funds was for "seeding" purposes, not to absorb the full costs of an HMO's development.
27. Dominick was an articulate, thoughtful conservative, who supported the HMO concept. He was not committed to AMA's stonewall position with regard to HMOs, but to a flexible federal commitment that would support a broad array of HMO prototypes, including fee-for-service, foundation plans.
28. Wayne Bradley, interview, Sept. 1974.

conservative medical establishment, forcing them to take an intransigent stance against HMOs:

> [Kennedy and Caper] deliberately assumed what we used to call in the labor movement, the opening to the left. [They] wanted to load up that bill with every conceivable kind of benefit that has some relationship to the needs of the public. And at least have a discussion of those issues.[29]

Intensive lobbying was not limited to the Congress. A concerted effort was made to pressure the Administration to reduce its heretofore unflagging enthusiasm for HMOs by prevailing upon White House staff to back away from the aggressively pro-HMO position of HEW. In early March 1972, AMA council members met with Richardson, who held firm to his commitment to the HMO strategy. John Iglehart, of the *National Journal,* reported at the time that at least one physician present at this meeting threatened to quit the President's reelection committee if this was the way physicians were to be treated by the Nixon Administration.[30]

The result of HEW's rebuff was to prod the AMA to pressure the White House directly. Malcolm Todd, M.D., chairman of the Physicians' Committee to Reelect the President, and a member of AMA's House of Delegates, complained to the President directly, in writing. Todd brought "all the force we could bring to bear" to get the Administration to back down on its HMO commitments.[31]

Then Rep. Gerald R. Ford (R-MI) was asked to call "an appropriate person in the executive branch," recommended by AMA staff, to express concern over the HMO commitment. Ford agreed to make such a call

---

29. James Doherty, interview, June 1974.

    It is interesting to speculate on whether AMA intransigence would have been mitigated had Sen. Kennedy not made his opening to the left. Based on AMA's initial position of conditional support for the Administration's experimental program, even though they saw no need for a categorical HMO assistance bill, it is likely they would have been much less vigorous in their counteroffensive had the debate been only between H.R.5615, the Administration Bill, and H.R.11728, the Roy-Rogers Bill. Without AMA intransigence, an HMO assistance bill would have cleared the 92nd Congress, since Rep. Rogers would have completed markup earlier in the session, allowing time for consideration by the full committee. AMA lobbyists take full credit for successfully delaying the markup and influencing full Commerce Committee Chairman Harley Staggers to drag his feet on the HMO bill.

30. John K. Iglehart. Health report/Intensive lobbying drive by medical group dims prospects for legislation. *Nat. J.* 4:1404, Sept. 2, 1972, AMA lobbyists have confirmed Iglehart's account and the one presented here.
31. *Ibid.*

and the lobbyists suggested that it ought to be made to Kenneth R. Cole, deputy assistant to Nixon for domestic policy, who was monitoring HMO activities for the White House.[32]

In a letter of thanks to Ford, Wayne Bradley, a coordinator of AMA's anti-HMO campaign on the Hill, noted:

> Your sympathetic consideration of the points we raised [at the meeting in your office] is greatly appreciated. As we indicated to you both before the meeting and at the meeting, it is not our intention to embarrass or feud with the Administration, but we believe that HMO strategy has the potential for serious problems.[33]

Paradoxically, James Cavanaugh, who had served as HEW's HMO policy coordinator for a short time in late 1970, was now a White House aide, charged with responsibility to calm the fears of the rank and file, largely Republican, AMA constituency.[34] At the AMA convention in June 1972, he assured the AMA membership that the Administration was not committed to anything more than a demonstration program.[35]

The timing of these White House responses to AMA overtures could not have been more embarrassing to Richardson, whose representatives were then involved in intense executive sessions with the House health subcommittee. Richardson made it clear that his and HEW's commitment to HMOs was unshaken.[36] However, the signals from the White House were much less enthusiastic and were read by wavering conservative Republican members as evidence that HMOs were not among the Administration's most burning priorities, as HEW had led them to believe. AMA tactics, in short, worked well in surfacing submerged, but

32. Wayne Bradley, "Ford Meeting," AMA internal memorandum, Mar. 20, 1972. This memorandum was part of a large file of confidential materials from AMA's Washington office, leaked to the press in 1975 by unknown parties. The details of the Ford approach on HMOs were first reported by Allan Parachini in the *Chicago Sun-Times*, July 23, 1975 ("Ford 1972 Pitch to White House for AMA Bared"). Parachini also noted the closeness of Ford to the AMA and observed that both the American Medical Political Action Committee (AMPAC) and the Michigan Medical Political Action Committee (MMPAC) had each contributed $2,500 to Congressman Ford's reelection campaign, a highly unusual move, inasmuch as such funds rarely went to safe districts.
33. Letter to the Hon. Gerald R. Ford from Wayne Bradley, Mar. 20, 1972. This letter was among the confidential AMA files leaked to the press in 1975.
34. AMA's White House lobbyist, Paul Donelan, was in almost daily contact with Cavanaugh on the HMO matter as the congressional debate heated up.
35. John K. Iglehart. Health report/Intensive lobbying drive by medical group dims prospects for legislation. *Nat. J.* 4:1404, Sept. 2, 1972.
36. Elliot L. Richardson, interview, June 1974.

always present, differences between the White House and HEW positions on HMO.

* * *

From the outset, White House commitments to HMOs had been of a different genre than those of HEW. Certainly, Domestic Council and OMB staff had endorsed the health maintenance strategy. But as the policy took on sharpened dimensions in the form of HMO assistance legislation, their commitment began to waver. White House staffers of the time steadfastly maintained that their position had never really changed; it just became more sharply defined as time went on.[37] HEW's position exceeded White House commitments to HMOs, especially after AMA made it clear to Cole and Cavanaugh that it was unhappy with the policy. By the summer of 1972, the gap between the White House and HEW had widened and become visible. Although HEW continued to advocate its program in congressional markup sessions, the message was filtering down from the White House to key minority members of the House Commerce health subcommittee that the real Administration position was much more conditional than the stated HEW position. At the same time, Richardson, outraged at press reports that he had knuckled under to AMA pressure, went out of his way to emphasize his personal commitment to HMO legislation by placing a number of phone calls to key subcommittee members, particularly to Rep. Harley Staggers, chairman of the full Commerce Committee, urging him to act favorably on the HMO bill.[38]

---

37. Kenneth R. Cole, who became staff director of the Domestic Council after John Ehrlichman's departure, had a very positive attitude toward HMOs. He had been involved in the 1970-71 policy process leading up to the Administration's commitment to HMO, was articulate in his knowledge about health care delivery system problems, and what HMOs might do to help solve them. Cole, however, insisted that the Administration's position had never been more than a commitment to demonstrate HMOs. HEW had gone too far, too fast, in its enthusiasm, and had made promises that could not be kept, requiring the White House to assert the true Administration position, beginning in 1972. Kenneth R. Cole, interview, Oct. 1974. Also, see chapter 3, pp. 63-64, for an account of Cole's efforts to place HMO on the Presidential agenda.
38. Secretary Richardson knew that the White House had lost its enthusiasm for HMOs and speculated that James Cavanaugh had been communicating directly with Republican members of the health subcommittee on the House side, letting them know that HMO was not of highest priority. But no direct pressure was brought to bear on Richardson himself to moderate his position. Cavanaugh, in fact, had called Chairman Staggers directly to articulate the White House's less than enthusiastic support for HMOs. In short, the House Commerce Committee was getting sharply conflicting guidance from the White House and HEW. They were articulating two different versions of Administration policy on HMO legislation.

The Administration had opened itself to the kinds of pressures it was now experiencing. The vacillation visible in mid-1972 was not merely the result of the AMA effectively applying pressure on the President and his staff. That was part of it. But other pressures were evident. HEW and the White House had never coordinated their efforts on health issues, so that throughout 1970 and 1971 no words of restraint, except perhaps during budget discussions, were ever conveyed to the Secretary. Even when it was apparent that the White House was attempting to lower its HMO profile, no restraints were placed upon Richardson. On the contrary, Ehrlichman had given him full responsibility for health policy formulation at their meeting in December 1970.

In a slightly different vein, HEW's zealous pursuit of its HMO policy throughout 1971 led to direct conflicts with other health constituencies over the tapping of PHS Act Section 314-e demonstration funds, RMP monies, and National Center for Health Services Research and Development Section 304 monies. Angered constituents of these programs lobbied the Public Health Service and their individual congressmen. And, as we have noted, AMA lobbyists pointed out to Rogers, Kennedy, and others that HEW was usurping congressional prerogatives by running an unauthorized HMO development program. Pressure on the Administration, in short, had been building steadily from other sectors of the health establishment (besides the AMA) and from congressional critics who resented the usurpation of their prerogatives. None of these pressures was designed to put HMOs in a favorable light.

The Senate Overcommits

The health community indicated varying degrees of support for Kennedy's bill, S.3327. Dominick of Colorado served as an articulate critic, both of the bill's nature and, especially, of the restrictive definition of an HMO found in Title I. During subcommittee markup in June, Dominick was not without sympathizers among his colleagues for his position, which would provide individual practice associations (IPAs) co-equal status with closed-panel groups.

Kennedy and Caper reacted to this rare show of independence by the usually passive health subcommittee by establishing a new category, called "supplemental HMOs," under Part B of Title I. Prepaid group practice HMOs, authorized in Part A, were still given priority status of funding; only if funds were left over after all available "true" (closed-panel, prepaid group practice) HMOs were funded could the Secretary of HEW fund supplemental HMOs. Title I, therefore, now (somewhat grudgingly) acknowledged the possibility that individual practice associations could be established in urban areas and not just relegated to rural areas, as under Title II. AAFMC had made some progress, although not nearly enough to satisfy them. In addition to rural "HSOs" there would now be "supplemental HMOs" — urban-based IPAs.

S.3327 was reported to the full Labor and Public Welfare Committee on June 15. No changes were made and the bill was reported to the Senate together with individual and minority views on July 21. Dominick voted to report the bill but took vigorous exception with the secondary status accorded to individual practice associations.[39] A possible conflict with the Finance Committee had been avoided by the elimination, during markup sessions, of the Health Maintenance trust fund, which would have required financing through a tap on federal cigarette and gasoline taxes. The Finance Committee discharged S.3327 without holding its own hearings.[40]

Meanwhile, AMA, having all but ignored Senate deliberations during subcommittee and full committee hearings, now made an all-out effort to kill S.3327. Kennedy, reacting to the apparent success of AMA in delaying full Senate consideration of his bill, launched a counteroffensive on August 17. In a news release and on the Senate floor, the senator from Massachusetts criticized organized medicine's attempt to bottle up S.3327: "This clumsy effort on their part is another example of the attempts of a narrow interest group to influence national legislation to its own advantage."

Again, on September 8, Kennedy appealed for consideration of his bill by the Senate. This time he sought to put pressure on the Administration to match its rhetorical commitment to HMOs with concrete support for Senate action. He noted again that the Administration was responding to AMA pressure and dragging its feet. Kennedy cited an article by the *National Journal's* Iglehart to bolster his claims. Iglehart noted that the Administration had reversed its position on the pre-emption of restrictive state laws issue. It had disclosed this new position at a closed markup session of the House bill on August 14. The new position was identical to the views on pre-emption expressed by the AMA.[41]

---

39. Report on S. 14, The Health Maintenance Organization and Resource Development Act of 1972, U.S. Senate, Committee on Labor and Public Welfare, Report No. 92-978.
40. Finance Committee Discharge of S.3327, *Congressional Record,* Aug. 1972.
41. AMA lobbyists had been meeting almost daily with White House staffer James Cavanaugh. The coincidence between the Nixon Administration's abrupt reversal on

The Senate finally took up S.3327 on September 20. The main activity centered around Dominick's efforts to amend the bill to cover IPAs co-equally with PPGPs. His amendment — Number 1447 — was vigorously debated, with significant support expressed. In the end, it was narrowly rejected, 37-40.

Dominick was not yet through, however. If Kennedy could not accept IPAs as co-equal, he could at least allow them a specific allocation of grant support: 25 percent of total awards. After hasty consultation on the Senate floor with Javits and Kennedy, Dominick agreed to accept a 17.5 percent allocation for supplemental HMOs. Kennedy reluctantly accepted the amendment, and S.3327 passed on September 20, by a 60-14 vote.

The Senate had given Kennedy and Caper virtually all that they asked for: a comprehensive bill with a $5.1 billion authorization. In the House, news of S.3327's passage with so sweeping a mandate disturbed supporters of HMO. At the same time, the news gave new hope to opponents of HMO. Both advocates and opponents knew that there was little prospect of a conference so late in the session between two bills so radically different in scope and purpose. The passage of S.3327, therefore, provided enemies of HMO all the ammunition they required to see to it that no HMO legislation passed the first session of the 93rd Congress.

The House Falters

Hearings on H.R.11728, the Roy-Rogers bill, and H.R.5615, the Administration's bill, did not begin until April 1972. Other pressing legislation kept HMO on a back burner for nearly six months, from the time it was first introduced in November 1971.

From the outset, the atmosphere in the House Health Subcommittee was very different from the Senate's. Here, HMO was viewed as an incremental reform, not as a total solution. Dominick's complaint that S.3327 was a large, promotional bill would have found much sympathy in the cautious and moderate House health subcommittee. Chairman Rogers signalled this cautious, deliberate approach in his opening statement:

---

pre-emption of restrictive state laws and AMA efforts at the White House level is evidence of the success of the medical organization's tactics. See: John K. Iglehart. Health report/Intense lobbying drive by medical group dims prospects for HMO legislation. *Nat. J.*, 4:1404, Sept. 2, 1972.

> HMOs . . . appear capable of becoming an integral part of our pluralistic health care delivery system, deserving of a chance to prove themselves through federal incentives. . . . The purpose of these hearings will be to determine the types and amounts of incentives which should be authorized, as well as explore the types of requirements which should be placed on HMOs receiving federal assistance. . . .[42]

The House health subcommittee hearings continued for 11 full days, concluding in May, and filling five volumes of testimony. Biles had, in the long months of crafting the House bill, touched base with virtually all of the major HMOs and health care interest groups in the country. Predictably, these organizations were brought forward to "make a public record" in favor of the Democratic alternative. There was some truth to the AMA charge that the hearings had been stacked in favor of the Roy-Rogers bill.[43]

Executive sessions extended from late May until September 21, when a clean bill, H.R.16782, was reported to the full Interstate and Foreign Commerce Committee. During that protracted period, five drafts of the bill were produced, the committee working primarily from H.R.11728, but scaling back the original Roy-Rogers bill with each successive draft.

The central issue in conflict was the scope of the grant program: would it be a large, multiyear program, supporting at least 250 projects, as Roy desired? Or would there be a 150 project limit, as the Republicans and conservative Democrats sought? The version reported to full committee authorized 150 projects, with a total spending authority of $335 million over a three-year period.

A second area of contention, effectively exploited by AMA lobbyists with conservative subcommittee members, was the "pre-emption of restrictive state laws" clause. Although every HMO bill contained a pre-emption clause, AMA lobbyists successfully induced the Administration to reverse its own position and to come out against pre-emption in August. The health subcommittee ultimately compromised on language designed to limit pre-emption to only the 150 projects funded under the federal act.

---

42. Paul G. Rogers, "Opening Remarks of the Chairman, Subcommittee on Public Health and Environment of the Committee on Interstate and Foreign Commerce," Hearings On Health Maintenance Organizations, Part I, U.S. House of Representatives, Apr. 1972, Serial No. 92-88, p. 2.
43. The hearings process is traditionally used to "make a public record" for a piece of legislation. Obviously, congressmen and their staffs, who have authorized a bill, will seek to put it forward in the best possible light.

The clean bill, H.R.16782, a greatly scaled down revision of H.R.11728, was reported to the full committee on September 21, one day after the Senate passed its $5.1 billion omnibus measure. Conservatives on the subcommittee, particularly Rep. Tim Lee Carter, M.D. (R-KY), and Rep. Ancher Nelson (R-MN), were being pressed very hard by the AMA. Their commitment to moving H.R.16782, therefore, was hardly enthusiastic and they privately expressed concern and doubts about the bill. The timing could not have been more inhospitable. Only a month was left until the fall elections and the prospect of a protracted conference with the Kennedy forces over so irreconcilable a match as their respective HMO bills was hardly welcome.

There was no great enthusiasm on the part of full committee Chairman Harley Staggers, either. He faced the difficult task of balancing priorities among four subcommittees and was genuinely undecided about what priority to assign to HMO in relation to other pressing bills. The chairman himself became the object of intense lobbying by forces for and against HMOs. On other occasions, Staggers could have relied on health subcommittee chairman Rogers to report only legislation that had the unambiguous and unanimous support of all health subcommittee members. The HMO bill was different. Even as Rogers was forging what he perceived to be a hard-won consensus, the intense lobbying efforts of the AMA were eroding it. By mid-September, these efforts were taking their toll so that H.R.16782 was reported only with the lukewarm support of influential Republican members Carter and Nelson. Nor was conservative Rep. David E. Satterfield III (D-VA) pleased with the bill, particularly the state override provision. In fact, he was the only member of the subcommittee to vote against clearing the bill to full committee.

Carter privately expressed his lack of enthusiasm for the HMO bill. The chief AMA lobbyist covering the Democrats, Howard Lee Cook, advised Staggers that he ought not move the bill with so short a time remaining in the session, particularly because the lobbyist had heard from a key Senate health subcommittee aide that Senate conferees would hold firm behind the core of S.3327. Moreover, Staggers was receiving conflicting signals from the Administration. James Cavanaugh, the senior White House health staffer, called Staggers and suggested that there was no great hurry on HMOs at about the same time that HEW Secretary Richardson was urging him to move the legislation out of committee.

Under these confusing circumstances, it was hardly surprising that Staggers decided to schedule other bills. He tabled H.R.16782 at the end of the 92nd Congress, where it died.

Consensus and Compromise

Although no HMO development legislation passed the 92nd Congress, each chamber turned quickly back to HMOs at the earliest possible time in the 93rd Congress. Kennedy reintroduced his already passed bill, S.3327, under the new number, S.14, on January 4, 1973. Roy and Rogers reintroduced their clean bill, H.R.16782, as H.R.51, on January 3.

The Administration introduced S.972 and H.R.4871, which represented a substantial retreat from its previous commitments, late in February. Through its new Secretary, Caspar W. Weinberger, HEW now declared its commitment to a limited, demonstration program, requested only a one-year, $60 million authorization, and deleted any reference to pre-emption of restrictive state laws.[44] The Administration's legislative position now reflected its lower rhetorical profile and dramatically illustrated the success of AMA's anti-HMO strategy.

As in the previous session, the Senate moved more quickly than the House, and S.14 passed on May 15. It was a substantially reduced version of the omnibus bill, S.3327. Again, the really protracted struggle took place in the House health subcommittee and the full Committee on Interstate and Foreign Commerce. Legislation successfully negotiated this arduous process and passed the full House on September 12.

* * *

Kennedy knew that he faced a different situation in his own subcommittee and on the Senate floor in 1973. In 1972, the width separating the Senate from the House on HMO assistance could only be approximated. Now, in 1973, it was all too clear how wide the gap was between the two branches. The Administration, moreover, had moved further to the right with its new bill, leaving Kennedy virtually alone in his enthusiastic support of a vast promotional effort. A $5.1 billion omnibus bill was just not going to sail through unchallenged and the senator instructed Caper to develop fallback positions in anticipation of expected challenges.

By the time Kennedy reported S.14 on April 7, 11 substantive changes had brought the bill down to a $1.5 billion, three-year authorization. Among the key changes made were broadened funding opportunities for supplemental HMOs; limitations on authorizations for annual quality health care initiative awards and capitation grant subsidies; Title V,

---

44. Letter of transmittal, H.R.4871, from Secretary HEW to Speaker of the House, Feb. 1973.

authorizing a National Institute of Health Care Delivery, was separated from S.14 and reported favorably as a separate bill. Then, each remaining section of S.14, authorizing an appropriation of funds, was amended to reduce funding levels.

Dominick was dissatisfied with these changes. He voted against reporting the bill favorably and filed a detailed dissent in the committee's report. Dominick declared:

> When the Committee reported S.3327 last year, I wrote individual views expressing in some detail my concerns with the approach that bill took. While this bill has been altered somewhat — pursuant to amendments I offered on the Floor last year and in Committee this year — its basic approach has not been significantly changed. Accordingly, my concerns remain essentially the same. I still feel this bill represents an attempt to promote one narrow form of health care delivery — closed-panel group practice — and that it would therefore limit the HMO concept's potential for improving our health care delivery system. I still think it is a mistake to encourage the development of delivery mechanisms, which can never be economically viable without continuing federal subsidies. I still believe the authorization levels are unrealistically high.[45]

On May 7, in anticipation of a fight for these principles on the Senate floor, Dominick filed three amendments, which, if passed, would radically scale down the scope of S.14. Then, on May 8, Sen. Robert Taft Jr. (R-OH) filed the Administration's bill, as an amendment to S.14. And, most ominous of all, two of Kennedy's most loyal supporters on the Republican side, Javits and Schweiker, filed, on May 9, a complete substitute amendment for S.14 — one that would have scaled the program back to $705 million over a one-year period.

S.14 clearly faced rough treatment from these five amendments. Kennedy and Caper plotted their own strategies, girding themselves in defense of their troubled proposal and also readying a number of fallback positions.

The debate began on May 14. Kennedy quickly dispatched the Administration's bill, offered by Taft in the nature of a substitute for S.14. He ridiculed the bill for its lack of specificity and for giving the Secretary "a blank check to do whatever he would like to do." The amendment was rejected.

---

45. "Minority Views of Senator Peter Dominick," Health Maintenance Organization Act of 1973, Report of the Committee on Labor and Public Welfare on S.14, Senate Report No. 93-129, Apr. 27, 1973.

The serious tests were yet to be encountered. Dominick called up his first amendment, which was a substitute for S.14. It proposed to delete provisions that he considered unworkable. These included elimination of grants for initial operating costs and increasing the amount of loans available for that purpose. Dominick also dropped special authorizations for rural health service organizations, area health education centers, capitation grants for the treatment of indigents and medically high-risk individuals, and subsidization of deficits incurred by operating HMOs. The Commission on Quality Health Care Assurance and special grants to health care institutions meeting quality standards were also deleted. The total price tag for Dominick's bill was $385 million.

Dominick argued persuasively that the President would veto any bill that resulted from a conference between the House and the Senate because the House health subcommittee had reported a bill authorized at only $280 million. He also noted that capitation grants for the poor were rightly part of an NHI program, not an HMO assistance bill.

Kennedy successfully fended off the Dominick attack on S.14, and the amendment fell by a 37-50 vote. Dominick then played his second amendment, which would have eliminated the capitation grants for subscribers with high-risk insurance ratings. Kennedy countered that this proposal would abandon lower-income families. Again he prevailed, but this time by only a 29-37 vote margin.

Dominick played his third and final amendment to eliminate only the quality assurance aspects of S.14. His amendment was dispatched by a vote of 40-47. However, Kennedy was shaken by the progressively narrowing gap on each successive vote on the Dominick amendments. He responded, finally, with his own substitute, cutting the authorization level to $865 million by eliminating separate authorizations for health service organizations and area health education centers. He also reduced authorizations for quality assurance and capitation grants by $355 million.

Kennedy's most significant concession was to give in on the important matter of co-equal status for IPAs. He dropped his three-tiered definition that discriminated between urban and rural, closed- and open-panel medical practice. This new position represented a decisive victory for AAFMC.

The Javits-Schweiker substitute amendment still remained to be answered, however, and, overnight, Kennedy cut a compromise with his two liberal Republican colleagues. On May 15, he withdrew his substitute of the previous day and submitted a new substitute, which, in effect, compromised the remaining differences between himself and Javits-Schweiker. Javits agreed to retain capitation grants for the poor but without a specific authorization. An earmark in the appropriation would suffice. Kennedy agreed to drop the medical malpractice program in S.14 and the Quality of Care Commission was moved into HEW rather than maintained with independent status. Javits's $705 million authorization level prevailed in the compromise.

The last substantive action on S.14, now significantly reduced from its original scope, was Sen. William D. Hathaway's (D-ME) amendment to add $100 million for rural HMOs. Hathaway agreed that his amendment was necessitated by the elimination of rural HSOs from S.14. The Senate agreed and supported the amendment by a vote of 80-14.

* * *

The nature of the House health subcommittee dictated a different turn of events than in the Senate. Whereas Kennedy's strong ideological and political control of his subcommittee meant that real challenges to S.14 could only be played out on the Senate floor, Rogers had to achieve consensus within his sharply divided subcommittee in order to have any chance of bringing legislation forward to the full Commerce Committee. The health subcommittee was only one of four subcommittees competing for attention on the full committee's crowded agenda and Chairman Staggers insisted that each subcommittee bring forward only those measures where substantial agreement had been achieved. Then, full committee efforts could be devoted primarily to procedural matters and minor technical amendments.

H.R.51 was the subject of two days of hearings on March 6 and 7. The new, limited demonstration approach of the Administration was praised by Rogers for its sensitivity to the prevailing viewpoint of his membership. Unlike in the Senate, the House health subcommittee sought to reconcile differences between its own bill, H.R.51, and the Administration's bill, H.R.4871. Rogers reported a clean bill, H.R.7974, on May 21.

The central issue during subcommittee deliberations was the number of projects to be assisted. Republicans urged a limit of 100 or fewer, while Roy insisted on support of at least 150. A compromise was fashioned that reduced the authorization level from $346.4 million to $280.7 million. The number of HMOs to be started with federal assistance was reduced from 150 to 100 for the first year of program operations, in an effort to come within the Administration's fiscal year 1974 budget figure.

H.R.7974, however, did not meet AMA or Administration objections to federally subsidized capitation (premium) supplements for low-income persons, nor did it limit the state override provision sufficiently. AMA lobbyists, therefore, continued working on subcommittee members in hopes of extracting further restrictions in the bill, and Rogers was pressed to reopen subcommittee markup sessions. Near the end of May, H.R.7974 was reconsidered by the subcommittee in several, sometimes heated, but unproductive sessions. By the July 4 recess, the bill was deadlocked in subcommittee. At issue were the capitation premium supplement for low-income families and the scope of the state override provision.

Over the July 4 recess, Rep. James F. Hastings (R-NY) and his aide, Spencer Johnson, came to Roy and Biles with the offer of a compromise, designed to bridge the gap between the liberal Democrats and conservative Republicans on the subcommittee. Roy and Biles readily agreed to the offer, and a so-called "Hastings compromise" was fashioned.

The Hastings substitute bill met 10 of 11 Administration objections to H.R.7974. It deleted the federal capitation supplement subsidy. It deleted the state override provision and modified the mandatory dual-choice provision so that it would apply only to employers with 25 or more employees.

The compromise was fashioned at two strategy meetings. The first involved just the two congressmen and their aides, Biles and Johnson. The second meeting involved representatives of GHAA, organized labor, and other interest groups, in order to gauge the chances for success if the compromise were to be introduced. It appeared to these strategists that the Hastings substitute for H.R.7974 would narrowly clear the full Committee on Interstate and Foreign Commerce, if brought up.

The health subcommittee formally met on the Hastings substitute about a week after the July 4 recess. HEW and the White House agreed to support the substitute. This satisfied the Republican members, who agreed to support the bill. By mid-July, Rogers was ready to go to full committee. Once again, as in the previous year, attention focused on Chairman Harley Staggers.

The year before, Staggers had been persuaded to let H.R.16782 die by not giving it a priority before the full committee. One AMA lobbyist even boasted that he had been instrumental in persuading the chairman not to take up the bill. A more reasonable explanation is that Staggers weighed and balanced all the forces at work, and concluded that other bills, showing greater consensus, should be given precedence.

In 1973, the big difference was the winning over of key Republican members to the Hastings compromise. This fact alone enabled Rogers to report out H.R.7974 a second time, with full subcommittee support. The question was how to get Staggers to take up the bill.

The answer came in the form of a request from GHAA's chief lobbyist James Doherty to Arnold Miller, United Mine Workers (UMW) president, for help in convincing Staggers of the importance of the HMO initiative. As a West Virginia congressman, Staggers was most responsive to his powerful mineworker constituency. Doherty briefed Miller on HMOs, and Miller met with Staggers. The UMW chief convinced the powerful chairman of the importance of H.R.7974 to his constituency and to the American people. Staggers, now convinced of the importance of HMOs, became an ardent supporter and promised to call up the bill promptly.

At this point, AMA made one last-ditch and foolhardy attempt to block consideration. H.R.7974 was scheduled for quick consideration by the full Committee on Interstate and Foreign Commerce on July 31, at 11:45 a.m., 15 minutes before it was to be brought to the floor of the House, where it clearly had the votes to pass. In a turbulent session, one committee member, prodded by AMA, called for a quorum. However, a quorum was not present, and the meeting terminated without consideration of the bill. The full House, therefore, was unable to vote on H.R.7974. Staggers was furious at so blatant a challenge to his prerogatives as chairman. He immediately scheduled committee meetings for the next three days and threatened to keep the committee in session around the clock, if necessary, until H.R.7974 received consideration.

Predictably, H.R.7974 received full committee attention on August 1. At this point, HMO advocates, who had urged consideration throughout the long summer of negotiations, now voiced objections to the size of the benefit package, which according to GHAA analyses, was just too expensive to permit the establishment of a competitive premium rate. Rogers's chief aide, Stephan Lawton, however, insisted that the bill be left intact. He had worked too hard to bring closure to the subcommittee's deliberations to allow the bill to be opened for reconsideration, at the 11th hour, in full committee.

H.R.7974 was adopted by voice vote on August 1 and reported out of committee on August 10. It authorized $240 million for grants, contracts, and loans to plan, develop, and initially operate HMOs over a five-year period. The bill passed the House on September 12, and the Senate bill, S.14, was adopted, substituting the language of H.R.7974.

The House demonstration approach clashed sharply with the $805 million promotional bill passed by the Senate three months earlier. The House-Senate conference, therefore, would — at long last — bring these two diametrically opposed approaches to federal HMO investment into direct confrontation.

The House-Senate Conference

The conference to reconcile differences between the House and Senate versions of the HMO assistance bills began in early November 1973 and concluded with a decisive compromise on the state override provision on November 28. The central issues were the low-income premium supplement, size of the benefit package, total numbers of HMOs to be authorized, the state override provision (in the Senate version), the mandatory dual-choice provision (in the House version), and quality assurance features from the Senate bill. In general, the conference adopted the House approach to HMO assistance, but retained significant features of the Senate bills. The result, as one observer has noted, was a "Cadillac chassis driven by a Volkswagen engine."

Low-income premium supplements were quickly discarded by the conferees, and it was agreed that the grant and loan program would be tailored to support about 100 projects over a five-year period. The conference settled on a benefit package somewhere between the expansive Senate requirements and the more modest House provisions. HMO industry representatives complained that, even with this compromise, it would be virtually impossible for plans to establish competitive rates, especially since premium supplements had been eliminated.

The House version of the mandatory dual-choice provision was also agreed to by Senate conferees. They had never opposed the provision, and had deleted it, only to placate organized labor. The adoption of a modified version of the state override provision, however, was controversial. In its final form, the provision could only apply to the 100 projects funded under the authorization of the bill. The four Republican conferees refrained from signing the conference report until they could see the exact final language. Eventually they signed the report, and House Report 93-714 on S.14 was filed on December 12. The House adopted the conference report by voice vote on December 18, with no debate. Senate action followed the next day, with only Sen. Herman E. Talmadge (D-GA) voting in opposition. Dominick of Colorado found the measure as passed quite acceptable.

P.L.93-222: How Workable?

Nixon signed the HMO bill on December 29, 1973. *In toto,* P.L.93-222 was a monument to the best in democratic politics and the worst in health care planning. The bill, as passed, retained open enrollment, community rating, and broad service package features far too cumbersome for the fragile HMO industry to handle in 1974. In the absence of financing provisions that would equalize the conventional health insurance industry's competitive edge, the combined effects of open enrollment, community rating, and service package would render plans' premium rates noncompetitive.

Feasibility of implementation, of course, was not foremost in the minds of the legislators responsible for the passage of P.L.93-222. Liberals, moderates, and conservatives each had their own, parochial motives as they pursued final passage of the act. As the final moments before closure approached, their true political agendas surfaced from behind the masks of public rhetoric:

- The state override provision was effectively exploited among conservatives as a states' rights issue. The usefulness of this argument for AMA was obvious: its overarching concern was to limit the role of the federal government in health and medical affairs.
- The mandatory dual-choice provision became a test of organized labor's control over the collective bargaining process.
- The scope of the mandated benefit package, open enrollment, and community rating divided pragmatic HMO industry advocates from utopian liberals in the Senate.
- The size of the federal assistance effort became the testing ground of organized medicine's ability to limit the scope of challenge to their hegemony. Their argument that HMOs should not get an unfair subsidy to compete against other forms of medical care failed to point out that fee-for-service medicine constituted a professional monopoly of awesome proportions, heavily subsidized by federal biomedical and (public/private) third-party vendor payment programs.
- The premium supplement debate involved the sensitive issue of the low-income health care consumer. Without the premium supplement, the HMO assistance bill had almost nothing to offer the poor. The subtle question of establishing a form of NHI through the back door was also raised by the premium supplement matter.

- Fiscal conservatives were temporarily separated from their traditional allies in organized medicine by the lure of HMOs' cost efficiency. The AMA's success in bringing fiscal conservatives back into their corner enormously boosted opportunities to water the bill down significantly.

The debate over HMO assistance cut to the core of contemporary health care politics. It jarred the power dynamics of the health establishment more keenly perhaps than the Medicare debate of a decade earlier. By exposing deep-seated tensions among delicately balanced health care components, HMO threatened, but also stimulated, the search for reform in health care systems. Faced with so awesome a challenge, HMO's enemies had only two choices: kill the federal initiative outright, or, failing that, shape the inevitable legislation in ways that would reduce its impact on established health care systems.

AMA, in particular, deserves high marks for its tactical successes in 1972 and 1973. In another sense, however, the strategy backfired because of the "foot in the door" hypothesis. Having now established the precedent of aggressive federal intervention in health care delivery systems, HMO advocates could set about to improve their law.

CHAPTER 7

The Limits of Health System Reform

The passage of Public Law 93-222, the HMO Act of 1973, was, in a sense, anticlimactic. Its arrival was so long overdue that the hard-won enthusiasm for HMOs generated in 1970 and 1971 had largely dissipated. The Nixon Administration succumbed early to the pressures of the medical establishment led by the AMA. By election time 1972, White House spokesmen were urging caution, and by early 1973, their retrenchment was complete: HMOs had become no more than demonstrations, and the Administration unenthusiastically proposed a limited three-year grant program.

The signals of 1972 and 1973 were clear enough to those who took the pulse of the nation's health politics: the word *demonstration* symbolized that the bloom was off the rose. HMOs would become just one more major health initiative launched with much hoopla and enthusiasm only to be consigned subsequently to bureaucratic obscurity. The health industry responded predictably. If the Administration had lost its enthusiasm for HMOs, the industry was certainly not going to stick its neck out. Thus, hospitals, physicians, health insurers, and related businesses began to turn away from HMOs after what had been an all too brief flirtation.

In late 1973, the enabling legislation had at last been enacted. But the climate of 1974 was markedly different from that of 1971. The Nixon Administration was in its final agonizing decline, and the early champions of HMO — HEW Secretary Elliot L. Richardson, Under Secretary John G.

Veneman, and Assistant Secretary for Planning and Evaluation Lewis H. Butler — had long since departed. Their successors were far less sympathetic to the HMO concept. Caspar W. Weinberger, the new HEW Secretary, was a Californian of a decidedly more conservative stripe than his predecessors. He was not an HMO advocate.

And in the Public Health Service, an inhospitable climate was to produce a sadly frustrated effort to implement the new HMO law.

1974-76: HMO Gets Lost in the Swamp — Again

The scale and complexity of the federal health bureaucracies are factors to be reckoned with in the search for national health policy. The health bureaucracies are collections of administrative fiefdoms, each with a narrow responsibility to subsidize or regulate a categorical element of the total health system. To reform the health system, therefore, one must also reform the federal health bureaucracies, which, at one and the same time, pursue and inhibit health system reform.

It is important to remember that implementation of the national HMO development program could occur only under the constraints and through the authority of the Public Health Service. Chapter 4 related how a major reorganization of the Health Services and Mental Health Administration (HSMHA) and other PHS elements, in 1973, was expected to impose the principles of functional management on the burgeoning array of categorical health programs that had proliferated over the past 15 years. The two objectives were to strengthen the managerial hand of the Assistant Secretary for Health and to improve the functional coordination among categorical programs. The immediate implication of this PHS reorganization for the revitalized HMO effort was to submerge the highly visible line agency Health Maintenance Organization Service (HMOS) into an obscure "program desk" within the newly formed Bureau of Community Health Services (BCHS), which, in turn, was a part of the Health Services Administration (HSA). This was accomplished during the summer and fall of 1973, well before Congress had authorized a substantial HMO program. Harold Buzzell, a private sector management consultant and friend of the new Assistant Secretary for Health, Charles Edwards, M.D., was the architect of the 1973 PHS reorganization plan. He became the director of HSA with direct authority over the HMO program.

When Gordon MacLeod resigned as HMO program director in protest over the 1973 reorganization, the somewhat thankless task of attempting to fulfill the new congressional mandate prescribed in the HMO Act of 1973 with less-than-adequate administrative tools at hand fell to Frank

1973 with less-than-adequate administrative tools at hand fell to Frank Seubold, Ph.D., an aerospace scientist from California, who had headed up the management division of the now defunct HMOS. In January 1974, Seubold was able to count on an operating staff of only six professionals, with most of the 50 former HMOS central office staff scattered among the five functional line divisions of BCHS. These personnel were available to the HMO program office only through a cumbersome and dysfunctional coordination process. Moreover, BCHS, as an organization, had virtually no understanding of the technical nature of HMO development and operations. Within the former administrative structure under HSMHA, the HMOS was able to develop an identity distinctive from the other PHS categorical programs. Now, as part of BCHS, that insularity disappeared: the HMO program office was only one small categorical activity among others that focused not on comprehensive health system reform, but primarily on specialized efforts to improve the health of the poor and medically underserved.

The situation was critical from the start. How could only six full-time central office professional staff members hope to reestablish a program that had been neglected for nearly two years (since the retrenchment of mid-1972)? There were regulations to be written and a grant program to launch. Many projects, funded during the pre-Act period, had been limping along with periodic infusions of nonmonetary technical assistance; now they required immediate direct financial subsidies if they were to move into operation.

The first order of business was to write and publish implementing regulations. Paul Batalden, M.D., the BCHS director, established several task forces to develop regulatory policy guidance. These task forces were staffed by his few full-time professionals, supplemented by expert temporary appointees, consultants, and health industry representatives. The task forces confirmed the worst fears of health industry representatives, particularly those representing the largest operating HMOs in the country. As they reflected on the precise meaning and interpretation to be applied to the new law, they began to realize just how inadequate P.L.93-222 was, from their point of view.

For example, if an operating plan wanted to avail itself of the opportunities for market development afforded by the mandatory dual-choice provision, it would have to become "qualified" within the meaning of Section 1310. This information startled the representative of one nationally known HMO. Until the task force experience, he had been unaware of the awesome power of the qualification requirement, which he now recognized as an unwarranted constraint upon his organization's economic independence.

In particular, the development of the Sub-Part H — Mandatory Dual-Choice regulation — illustrated the complexity faced by those trying to work with the new law. The concept would require employers subject to the provisions of the Fair Labor Standards Act of 1938 to offer the HMO as a health benefits option where qualified plans were available. This idea had originally been suggested by the American Rehabilitation Foundation and accepted by Brian Biles and Philip Caper, aides to Rep. William R. Roy (D-KS) and Sen. Edward M. Kennedy (D-MA), respectively, in drafting House and Senate versions of the HMO enabling act. The provision had been deleted from the Senate bill, S.14, after organized labor objected that it would seriously infringe its collective bargaining rights.[1] As it turned out, labor's fears were entirely justified. The provision carried into law reflected essentially the House language and soon ran afoul of Public Health Service legal interpretations.

Assistant General Counsel Sidney Edelman was called upon to interpret the mandatory dual-choice provision. Edelman chose a literal and narrow interpretation: in his opinion, Section 1310 intended that each individual employee must be allowed to choose an HMO if the option were available in his area, even if a collective bargaining agent had already rejected the HMO plan in contract negotiations with management. Technically, Edelman was correct: the Fair Labor Standards Act of 1938 established employee rights to a minimum wage. If HMO health benefits were available under the protection of the minimum wage act, then those rights were mandatory and could not be abrogated by a collective bargaining agreement.

In protecting an individual employee's right to choose an HMO option, however, HEW was abrogating provisions of the National Labor Relations Act of 1935 that also protect workers, but through a different right, the right to organize into labor unions and to bargain collectively for wages and benefits. The Fair Labor Standards Act protected workers as individuals, while the National Labor Relations Act enabled them to take collective action for their mutual benefit. The PHS Assistant General Counsel argued that the literal meaning of Section 1310 required the National Labor Relations Act collective bargaining provision,

---

1. HMO lobbyists clearly sought as flexible an interpretation of the 1310 authority as possible. In particular, they wished to reserve for HMOs the right to market directly to employees, even when a collective bargaining agent had specifically opted not to offer the HMO option as part of a union's health benefits package. Labor representatives had been apprised of the HMO lobbyists' position and had not initially objected. However, their national councils took vigorous exception to this position.

protecting the unions' hard-won right to act as sole agents for their members, to recede before the more pressing right of the individual's access to an HMO plan.

Organized labor denounced the PHS interpretation. When the notice of proposed rule making (NPRM) was published in February 1975, the Secretary of Labor and the National Labor Relations Board both filed official objections. Indeed, Weinberger wisely acceded to the labor movement and Sub-Part H was substantially revised prior to publication, in final form, in the fall of 1975. And to avoid any further ambiguity, the HMO Amendments of 1976 added a provision to Section 1310 requiring that, where a collective bargaining agent was present, he must first be presented with the offer to market an HMO. The agent's decision to offer or not to offer the HMO option to union members would be considered binding.

The two years' delay in clarifying Section 1310 significantly impeded HMO development. Businesses were not about to establish HMO benefit plans until the collective bargaining status of labor was clear. Many potential HMO developers shied away from the program because they would not be able to take advantage of the marketing opportunities afforded by mandatory dual-choice until regulations had been promulgated.

Similarly, the prospective reimbursement provision under Section 1876 of the Social Security Act was virtually useless as an incentive for generating substantial enrollments of Title XVIII (Medicare) recipients in HMOs. Before July 1, 1978, there were only 25,000 persons enrolled in HMOs under Section 1876, and only 16,000 of these were enrolled under the at-risk provisions governing the reimbursement of "established" HMOs. The remaining 9,000 were enrolled under the cost-reimbursement provision governing new HMOs.[2]

When the HMO development program set about to stimulate new HMO activity, it was frustrated and encumbered by a bureaucratic structure unworkable from inception, a regulatory environment displaying a decided lack of sensitivity to the needs of a struggling new program, and a Republican Administration that had long since lost its appetite for health system reform. All this, and a law to implement that was adjudged by knowledgeable industry representatives to be unrealistically demanding in its multiple requirements for broad benefits, open enrollment of membership, and community rating of premiums.

---

2. See chapter 5, pp. 95-106, for a discussion of the "at-risk" and "cost" reimbursement mechanisms.

Not surprisingly, the progress of HMO development was slow throughout 1974, 1975, and 1976. Not only were all the foregoing obstacles endured, but the national economy experienced its worse recession in 20 years, coupled with continued and unrelenting double-digit inflation. Under the best of circumstances, it was not an auspicious time to stimulate substantial new developmental efforts in the private health economy.

Congress, however, was willing to spend money to develop new HMOs. By the time the HMO Development Office was nearing completion of interim regulations governing disposition of the grant and loan programs, Congress had passed a supplemental appropriation of $25 million for grants and contracts. This was followed, soon after the beginning of fiscal year 1975, by a regular appropriation of $15 million. Thus, the first official post-Act grant rounds had a sizable budget of $40 million available for distribution.

Congress is a fickle ally, at best. The subtleties and extraordinary difficulties of bureaucratic management are, for the most part, lost in the legislative process. Having struggled for three years to produce a piece of HMO legislation, the members of the authorizing committees were eager to see solid and measurable results. Moreover, having passed the supplemental appropriations for HMOs, the appropriations committees now expected a program of sufficient scale and scope to justify their lavish support. Failure to meet congressional expectations would most certainly be harshly received in subsequent oversight hearings and appropriations reviews.

The problem was to find qualified recipients — not an easy assignment since the HMO development effort had been at a virtual standstill since mid-1972. After the first two preoperational grant rounds, the resourceful HMOS staff had established six resource development contracts with national organizations in the hope that they would stimulate significant HMO development among their memberships. These contracts produced few new HMOs, however, so that after nearly three years the program could point to no unique development experience directly related to federal efforts.

Now, as the HMO program office geared up for a new round of grant activity, it lacked virtually all of the vehicles for success. It had almost no central office staff. It was housed in a bureau with no professional understanding or capability to implement a program as complex as HMO. And its potential clients in the communities were not primed for a sustained HMO development effort.

The regional office situation was particularly unpromising. The PHS regional offices were the first, and practically only, channel of communication between HEW and the community to be served by federal investments. Buzzell, the HSA administrator, had issued a memorandum, in February 1974, requesting that the 10 regional health administrators make a major staff commitment to full-time HMO work. Buzzell's request was only partially fulfilled by regional officials, who, under the functional scheme of organization established in 1973, reported directly to the Assistant Secretary for Health, not to the HSA administrator. Staff professionals, moreover, were responsible for multiple program areas inasmuch as they, too, were organized along functional, not program area, lines. Thus, there was no easy way for the HMO program office in the HSA/BCHS to get regional office cooperation. The result was that regional office staff members were available only about 75 percent of the time, at most, for HMO matters. In many regions, this percentage was never even approached. Moreover, HMO central office staff could not supervise their work directly. It was a hopeless administrative predicament.[3]

Beyond that, regional office cooperation depended on the conviction that a grant appropriation would be forthcoming. In 1974, the sad experience of two years earlier still haunted the central office HMO program staff. In March 1972, HSMHA Administrator Vernon E. Wilson, M.D., had instructed the regional offices that the third pre-Act grant round had been cancelled and that already approved projects could not be funded. This time, the regional offices would take no chances: only when Congress approved an appropriation and the Office of Management and Budget (OMB) had released the funds for use would they begin to stimulate applicant interest.

The results of the first grant round, in the summer of 1974, were predictable: there were only 125 applications nationally, and fully one-half of these were unacceptable, displaying virtually no understanding of

3. The General Accounting Office presented a very negative report to the Congress on HEW's management of the HMO effort. GAO focused its criticisms on HEW's functional reorganization plan of 1973, which had fragmented responsibility for HMO program management among many organizational units. See: U.S. Senate, Committee on Labor and Public Welfare. Subcommittee on Health. 94th Congress. Hearings on S.1926 Health Maintenance Organization Amendments 1975. November 21, 1975, December 12, 1975, January 19, 1976. Washington DC: U.S. Government Printing Office,1976. Also see: U.S. Senate. HMO Amendments of 1976. Report from the Committee on Labor and Public Welfare on S.1926, May 13, 1976, Report No. 94-844. Washington, DC: U.S. Government Printing Office, 1976.

the complexities of HMO development. The second grant round, begun late in the fall, confirmed the trend: no qualified applicants were forthcoming. In all, five grant rounds were required in fiscal year 1975 in order to squeeze out 375 applications. By the summer of 1978, the status of the 158 applicants funded in fiscal 1975 was as follows: 45 (29 percent) were qualified HMOs, 35 (27 percent) were still actively pursuing development, and 78 (49 percent) were inactive or defunct.

The HMO program office spent only $22.5 million of the $40 million appropriated by the Congress in fiscal years 1974 and 1975. Even so, the HMO program was criticized because of the apparent low quality of many of the approved projects. This problem was directly related to the faulty administrative structure of the program, that is, limited central office personnel, inadequate regional office effort, and a fragmented functional bureaucratic base.

The separation of the "qualification" and "regulatory compliance" functions from the "development" function, a direct result of interpretations applied to the enabling act and implemented through the 1973 PHS reorganization, graphically illustrated HEW's inept management of the HMO effort to the General Accounting Office (GAO) and congressional oversight committees.[4] The subsequent lack of coordination between the development and qualification offices was cited by both the GAO and the Office of the Assistant Secretary for Health (OASH) as a major reason for difficulties experienced by the PHS in its implementation of the HMO act.[5] In particular, the OASH review faulted the qualification review process for failing to communicate effectively with the development program. The result was a serious bottleneck at the point when developing projects became operational and sought qualification under the provisions of Section 1310. By early 1977, the backlog had grown to over 50 operational plans awaiting review of their applications for qualification.

Because the HMO development program had difficulty finding qualified new projects during the first two fiscal years under the enabling act authority, Congress appropriated no more than the Administration's request for fiscal year 1976. In the opinion of OMB and the HEW Office of the Secretary, this funding request was entirely consistent with a five-year demonstration program. On the assumption that the program would not be renewed after the five-year period, only sufficient funds were re-

---

4. *Ibid.*
5. *Ibid.*

quested to support projects already in the development "pipeline" and for enough "new starts" so that the pipeline would close down by the end of five years. Thus, OMB's plan was to allow *feasibility studies, planning, initial development* and *loans* for the first three years; only *initial development* and *loan* support in the fourth year; and, finally, only *loans* in the fifth year.

This approach was unworkable because it ignored the usual administrative practice of anticipating amending legislation to continue categorical health programs beyond their initial authorizations, an accepted practice during earlier Democratic administrations. It was also unworkable because it displayed no understanding of the developmental nature of HMO projects. Unlike traditional PHS subsidy projects, which were operational almost from their inception, HMOs could not traverse their arduous developmental course unless they received critically spaced, and progressively larger, infusions of working capital until they became operational. Then the loan programs would take over until a break-even point was achieved when premium revenues to cover expenses equalled incurred costs. Moreover, the front-end cost of HMO development was high: some estimates placed the average costs at $5 million before the breakeven point could be achieved, three to five years into operations.

The Office of the Secretary/OMB funding plan completely ignored these basic facts about HMO development. HMOs were business enterprises, not welfare-like subsidy programs, a notion not well understood in the HEW Secretariat of 1974-76.

Increasingly harsh congressional criticism of HEW's management led to the abandonment of the byzantine functional management of the HMO program in BCHS, in November 1975. The new Assistant Secretary for Health, Theodore Cooper, M.D., instructed HSA to consolidate all HMO development activities within a single line agency. The activity was transferred from BCHS to the Bureau of Medical Services, as the Division of HMO Development (DHMOD), with five branches. The program's fortunes now began to improve. An unexpected windfall resulted from the change in fiscal year from July to October, bringing in an additional $4 million to cover operating costs for this one-time "transition quarter." And during the summer of 1976, a new HSA administrator, Louis Hellman, M.D., allowed the DHMOD to take an appeal for a supplemental appropriation directly to Cooper. The request, bottled up for nearly a year in an unsympathetic HSA, was immediately approved by Cooper, and a $3.8 million second grant round supplemental request was prepared for congressional review. The funding picture for fiscal year 1976 appeared as follows:

$15.0 million	FY 1976 appropriation
$ 4.0 million	Transition quarter appropriation
$ 3.8 million	Supplemental appropriation
$22.8 million	Total budget

However, HEW's controller failed to transmit the supplemental appropriation request to the House appropriations committee until September 15. Because this gave the congressional appropriations committee only two weeks to consider the request, not surprisingly, it refused to honor it.

The final fiscal year 1976 appropriation was only $19 million. The second cohort of grantees, already approved for funding, was told that the award cycle had been cancelled. The impact on the private sector of potential HMO developers was, according to one thoughtful observer, "devastating." The effect on PHS regional office staff was demoralizing: for the second time in less than four years, they had trusted Washington, only to be embarrassed with their constituents and clients in the states and communities. The events of fiscal year 1976, therefore, were pivotal. Any hope that HEW, under a Republican Administration, would undertake a serious and vigorous HMO development program was lost in the mire of bureaucratic indirection.

The Administration's intentions were confirmed in the fiscal year 1977 budget negotiations: OMB instructed HEW to request no additional funds for HMO feasibility studies. The game plan would be played out. A terminal five-year effort was all that would be tolerated.

* * *

It would be the ultimate in understatement to describe the feelings of committed HMO advocates as unhappy. *Dismayed* would be a more appropriate word. The combination of a restrictive enabling act, determined obstruction at the highest levels of the Ford Administration, and the inevitable bureaucratic inertia that develops when top-level policy makers let a program fend for itself within a hostile administrative environment — all these factors weighed heavily on HMO advocates. Their early experiences with the PHS regulatory drafting mechanisms also convinced them that their only hope was to seek relief through the Congress. And so, the HMO consensus group was created.

The HMO Consensus Group: Lobby for Change

Prior to the passage of P.L.93-222 in December 1973, the lion's share of lobbying advocacy had been by the Group Health Association of America, led by its legislative director, James Doherty. Only rarely during the three years of pre-Act legislative struggle was there any effort to coordinate lobbying activities among all of HMO's major advocates. Gordon MacLeod, M.D., the director of HMOS, had assembled an informal advisory group, with which he met periodically in 1972 and 1973 to gain insights on both legislative and administrative issues. And from time to time, informal, confidential meetings were held between key congressional and administrative staffers, under the auspices of leading HMO advocates. The informality of those meetings immeasurably aided in the coordination of legislative strategies, in ways that could not have been accomplished through more formal channels. These are commonplace events in the legislative process, where lobbyists often provide important vehicles of communication for formal actors in the system, who normally do not — often, because they cannot — talk to one another.

A formal coalition of HMO advocates, however, had not emerged from these episodic gatherings and encounters. Nevertheless, by December 1973, most of the players in the HMO saga knew one another, and, for the most part, were on a friendly basis. The passage of P.L.93-222 provided a common framework for these advocates to work together. Their motivation was the nearly unanimous conviction that the law, as written, was unrealistic in its expectations and unworkable in practice.

Meeting with HMO staff in the PHS, during the winter of 1974, provided a natural point of congregation for the advocacy groups. A milestone was reached when, following a meeting of the Health Insurance Association of America, the influential Blue Cross Association, as well as leading indemnity carriers such as Aetna and Connecticut General, decided not to oppose the Section 1310 provision. The insurance industry, in short, decided not to oppose the legal basis through which HMOs could challenge their heretofore undisputed dominance of local health care markets. This was the final obstacle to achievement of a fundamental consensus. If the insurers could accept the struggling prepaid plans in the competitive marketplace, all other points of contention could be resolved. A united front could be presented to the Congress.

The HMO consensus group — composed of GHAA, Blue Cross Association, American Group Practice Association, American Association of Foundations for Medical Care, some individual insurers, a number of established HMOs, and the Health Insurance Association of

America — met frequently in the latter months of 1974 and into the winter of 1975. During that time, consensus was achieved on a dozen amendments. The focus was on three aspects of the law that were particularly obnoxious to the established plans.

First, the consensus group sought elimination of mandated benefits not originally specified in pre-Act requirements. They proposed to make the provision of home health services, radiological services, and associated laboratory fees optional. Mental health and alcoholism services were retained as part of the required outpatient mix because the consensus group was not about to take on the powerful mental health lobby.

Second, the consensus group sought to delete the open enrollment requirement. Under the statutory language passed in 1973, a qualified HMO had to open its enrollment each year for at least a period of 30 days to all comers, on a first-come, first-served basis. The problem with this requirement was that HMOs expected to derive the bulk of their new enrollees from organized employer-employee groups, which could deliver large and stable enrollments. The planned marketing of these groups, coupled with projections of total enrollment capacities, was a significant element in an HMO's long-term planning. Open enrollment challenged the principle of prudent market planning. An unpredictable number of individual enrollees could walk through the doors, upsetting growth projections dependent upon marketing programs directed toward organized groups. In short, open enrollment, a concept that in theory promotes equity of access, could seriously disrupt the structured, disciplined marketing efforts of prepaid health plans and render actuarial and cost projections meaningless.

Beyond these issues, P.L.93-222 tied open enrollment to community rating. The two approaches taken in tandem offered a deadly combination. The unpredictable enrollment, during an open-enrollment period, of individuals who could only be charged premiums based on the single community rate, promised to disrupt the delicate balance between enrollment projections, the establishment of rates, and the overall fiscal integrity of the plan. The spectre of high-risk individuals enrolling at standard community rates during the open enrollment period was a frightening possibility. Community rating might be endured, but not in tandem with open enrollment. An HMO had to be allowed to control its risks.

With the amendments ready to·go by the spring of 1975, a legislative strategy had to be devised. One thing was certain: the House would be the initial focus of the effort. It was essential to introduce amendments in the

House and move the process as far as possible in that body, before action began in the Senate. The House amendments had to set an appropriate standard for the Senate. Certainly, under Caper's and Kennedy's watchful eyes, there could be little hope of active support for the consensus group's proposed amendments in the Senate, although Kennedy and Caper were not expected to block consideration.

Then, too, the AMA was expected to oppose the "consensus" amendments. Knowing that the law as passed was unworkable, AMA embraced the opportunity to strike a pose in favor of "equity" and "social justice," resisting any changes that would scale it down to encourage more effective implementation. AMA was committed to seeing HMOs fail.

The consensus group strategy, then, was first to put the bill through the House, while isolating the antiamendment positions of Kennedy and the AMA. Early in the spring, Spencer Johnson, Rep. James Hastings's aide, called Jim Doherty at GHAA. Hastings was proud of the pivotal role he had played in 1973 in fashioning the decisive compromise between conservatives and liberals on the House health subcommittee. Hastings and Johnson were looking for ways to reassert their leadership in the HMO policy arena, and Johnson expressed an interest in proposing amendments. Doherty, of course, was ready to respond positively to the call, and he summarized the results of the consensus group's efforts. Johnson was impressed with what he heard — particularly the fact that broad agreement had been reached on a common set of amendments by all key interest organizations in the HMO industry.

At a meeting between the consensus group and Hastings, the congressman agreed to seek cosponsorship for the amendments with subcommittee chairman Rep. Paul G. Rogers (D-FL). These activities were observed with interest by Sen. Richard S. Schweiker (R-PA), who had long believed that the 1973 HMO act was detrimental to HMO growth and development. He reviewed the proposed House amendments and agreed to cosponsor their introduction in the Senate, if organized labor concurred with them. Schweiker received assurances of labor's sympathy.

On June 12, 1975, Hastings and Rogers introduced H.R.7847, the HMO Amendments of 1975, in the House, while Schweiker, with Sen. Walter F. Mondale (D-MN) as cosponsor, introduced an identical bill, S.1926, on the same day. The approach to Mondale was particularly ingenious. Kennedy, through Caper, had agreed to keep an open mind about the amendments. But, since most of the proposed changes would undo features of the bill rooted in Caper's and Kennedy's determination to tie substantial health system reforms to the HMO act, they could not be counted upon to embrace the amendments enthusiastically. Hence, it was particularly appropriate for Paul Ellwood, the original HMO proponent, now president of InterStudy, successor organization to the American Rehabilitation Foundation, to enlist the support of Mondale, one of his home state senators. Other liberal members of the Senate health subcommittee were effectively lobbied by well-established HMOs from their home states.

In short, the HMO amendments had broad support in the Senate health subcommittee, even as they were introduced. Kennedy and Caper faced the virtual certainty of amendment. They would now be forced to try to shape those amendments so as to produce the least erosion to the original concepts they had included in P.L.93-222. Their role now would be defensive and reactive.

The HMO Amendments of 1976: A More Workable Law Emerges

The initiative for change was in the House. Key backers of the original bill had always harbored doubts that the expansive bill finally agreed to, through the 1973 conference committee compromise, could ever work, stripped as it was of the lavish funding provisions originally proposed by Kennedy. Hastings, in particular, was eager to undo the harm of the past two years, and he prevailed on Rogers to schedule early hearings.

These came on July 14 and 15, 1975. As drafted, H.R.7874 would allow HMOs to offer so-called supplemental services at their option, not at the patients' options; it would make treatment and referral services for alcohol and drug abuse, home health services, and preventive dental care for children optional supplemental services instead of required basic services.

The bill would also drop the open-enrollment requirement, delay the community rating requirement for five years, and delete provisions requiring HMO physicians in group practice to devote at least 50 percent of their time to HMO work. Authorizations would be extended for two years. Organized labor, reacting strongly to HEW's decision to press forward with final dual-choice option regulations that would force an employer to offer an HMO option to employees, even though it had been rejected by a collective bargaining agent, offered language mandating the collective bargaining agent the right to first offer and refusal of the HMO option.

The hearings documented the slow implementation of HMO development under HEW's complicated PHS management structure. There were no serious objections to consensus group proposals, except those voiced by AMA. The AMA's principal complaint was that the amendments would subvert the intent of P.L.93-222 by eliminating the very provisions that would have demonstrated whether or not HMOs could provide comprehensive health care at reasonable cost. Why offer federal subsidies to organizations not proposing to attempt unique and innovative means for delivering health care?

AMA's sudden concern for the purity of the HMO experiment was particularly disingenuous, coming so soon after its all-out assault on the original legislation. By blocking amendments, AMA proposed to ensure the continued unworkability of the federal HMO program. Hastings noted at the time, "It's plain to me that they're opposed to HMOs and would like to see them go down the tubes." Schweiker concurred: "It's another way to ax it."[6]

One week after the close of hearings, on July 23, the House Interstate and Foreign Commerce Committee health subcommittee finished its markup and reported out a clean bill, H.R.9019, to the full committee. Each of the key provisions supported by the consensus group remained intact, except that home health services were retained as a basic benefit.

The HMO Amendments of 1975 were reported by the full subcommittee on September 26, 1975, with virtually no changes from the subcommittee report. Rep. Tim Lee Carter, M.D. (R-KY), and Rep. David E. Satterfield III (D-VA), generally sympathetic to AMA views, repeated protests made in subcommittee. They offered the only dissenting and supplemental views: principally, that P.L.93-222, as originally passed, ought to be given its full three-year test and evaluated. H.R.9019 proposed to "change the rules in the middle of the game."[7]

* * *

The Senate was another matter. Kennedy, as we have noted, expressed no real enthusiasm for the prospect of amendment. While promising to keep their minds open, Kennedy and Caper were deeply committed to some of the elements of the original legislation that the consensus group and a number of other senators now believed were inhibiting HMO development. But the lead was Schweiker's. He had vainly sought a more modest and scaled-down Senate bill in 1972 and again in 1973. Deter-

---

6. Remarks of Rep. James Hastings and Sen. Richard S. Schweiker, quoted in the *Congressional Quarterly*, Aug. 9, 1975, p. 1775.
7. Rep. Carter, however, voted for the amendments — an interesting example of speaking out on one side of his political mouth while voting out of the other.

mined minorities of one period are often the harbingers of future majorities, particularly when intervening events support their views. So it was for Schweiker. The dismal experience of HMO development in the two years under P.L.93-222 spoke clearly to the need for a legislative remedy.

Kennedy opened hearings on the proposed amendments in late November, four months after the House had heard testimony. His opening statement made it clear that, for his part, the slow progress under P.L.93-222 should be laid at HEW's doorstep. Schweiker, however, focused on the shortcomings of the Act, emphasizing that, under P.L.93-222, HMOs could not compete effectively in the health care marketplace.

S.1926 was identical to H.R.9019, providing six basic modifications to P.L.93-222:

- An identifiable, staffed unit in HEW to administer the HMO program and to get the program moving rapidly and effectively
- Changes in the benefit package to allow certain services to be transferred from basic to supplemental, so that HMOs could compete in cost terms with more conventional insurance schemes
- Provisions for phasing in both the health services and the enrollment of prepaid members, to facilitate the start-up of HMOs in communities that have not had the opportunity to identify with these new forms of health care delivery
- Clarification of the dual-choice provisions to ensure that the decision respecting health care coverage options in employer-employee relations would continue through the collective bargaining process
- Relieving HMOs from the requirement of providing an open-enrollment period, a requirement not imposed on other health insurance schemes
- Strengthened provision for assistance loans and loan guarantees to HMOs that serve medically underserved populations

The General Accounting Office had conducted a preliminary evaluation of experience under P.L.93-222 during its first 1½ years. Its findings tended to support the main thrusts of H.R.9019 and S.1926. Substantial majorities of operating HMOs agreed that the expansive benefits, open enrollment, and community rating requirements would tend to make HMOs noncompetitive.

Kennedy and Caper were willing to accept the notion that the Act, as originally passed, was too expansive. But Caper was adamant about retaining a meaningful open-enrollment provision. Thus, Kennedy and his aide moved S.1926 swiftly through the subcommittee by reserving debate over open enrollment until full committee markup. The real battleground was the full committee, during the spring of 1976.

The HMO consensus group, anticipating the coming struggle over open enrollment, solicited the help of the chairman of the full Labor and Public Welfare Committee, Sen. Harrison A. Williams Jr. (D-NJ), through the good offices of a number of successful and influential New Jersey-based HMOs. Williams's aide, Nick Eddis, drafted a compromise open-enrollment position. Caper had been holding firm on a "10 percent of net new enrollment" position.[8] The consensus group still held out for total elimination of the proposal, the House position. Eddis came up with a proposal for open enrollment of 4 percent of net new enrollment annually. Significantly, the definition of net new enrollment excluded new members coming in through existing employee group contracts. This meant that new enrollees, coming in through the large Federal Employees Health Benefits Program and local union contracts, would not be included in the calculation. The consensus group was very pleased with the Williams compromise. It went beyond their most optimistic hopes.

Caper would not accept the Williams compromise. Shortly before the final markup session, the HMO consensus group, accompanied by an influential representative of organized labor, made a last effort to budge Caper on open enrollment. The meeting failed in this objective. Kennedy's position would be to solve the open-enrollment problem from the other end of the spectrum: since the arguments against it were that open enrollment did not apply equally to the health insurance industry, Kennedy would offer an amendment to apply the concept to the entire health insurance industry!

The senator from Massachusetts did just that: he offered his amendment at the full committee markup in early May 1976. His colleagues were flabbergasted. Mondale humorously suggested that they adjourn the session to the Capital Centre (Washington's large sporting and convention facility), because "some" insurance industry representatives might have some things to say. Schweiker suggested that the proposal was completely outside of the Committee on Labor and Public Welfare's jurisdiction. Kennedy realized, at this point, that he and Caper had reached the outer limits of, and perhaps had gone beyond, a reasonable defense of open enrollment. He called for a test vote on his controversial amendment and was defeated 10-5.

---

8. This meant that an HMO would have to increase its enrollment by a minimum of 10 percent of the previous year's average new enrollment.

Williams, at this point, introduced his compromise proposal, which the committee accepted. The "4 percent" figure was compromised down to "3 percent" in the Senate-House conference. Kennedy filed "additional views," along with Sen. Gaylord Nelson (D-WI) and Sen. William D. Hathaway (D-ME), at the time the bill was favorably reported:

> If there is any validity to the argument that the unilateral imposition of an open-enrollment requirement on HMOs and not other health care insurers places HMOs at a competitive disadvantage, we would have preferred to see the committee deal with it by imposing open-enrollment and community-rating requirements on the entire health insurance industry, including HMOs.
>
> In our view, elimination of the open-enrollment provision represents a giant step backwards in terms of federal health policy in this country.[9]

The course was already set, however. In a rare show of independence from Kennedy's leadership, the Williams amendment on open enrollment passed with other provisions relaxing the strictures of P.L.93-222.

The Committee on Labor and Public Welfare reported S.1926 to the Senate on May 13, 1976. The Senate took up the measure on June 14. The only real controversy was Kennedy's announcement that he would vote against the bill because of the open-enrollment limitation. The breadth of committee support for the measure, however, ensured passage.

The House-Senate conference was held on September 13 and generally took a middle ground on those issues where the House and Senate differed. The House conferees agreed to retain the framework of the Senate position on open enrollment. Under the conference agreement, HMOs that had been in business for at least five years or enrolled more than 50,000 persons would have to open their enrollment for a 30-day period annually, if they were financially viable. However, the number of persons enrolled through this mechanism would not have to exceed 3 percent of the total increase in enrollment during the previous year. Senate conferees dropped their 4 percent requirement in favor of the 3 percent figure. Significantly, the conferees retained the definition of *net new enrollment,* to be based upon enrollment under new contracts, exclusive of members coming in through existing contracts.

---

9. U.S. Senate. HMO Amendments of 1976. Report from the Committee on Labor and Public Welfare on S.1926, May 13, 1976, Report No. 94-844. Washington, DC: U.S. Government Printing Office, 1976, p. 32.

The community rating provision, argued the HMO consensus group, put HMOs at a competitive disadvantage with conventional health insurance plans that experience rated. The House had moved to waive the requirement for all HMOs for up to five years. The Senate, however, distinguished between new HMOs and existing HMOs. Existing HMOs would be required to comply with community rating requirements, whereas new plans could have up to three years to comply. The Senate had also insisted that the waiver apply only to basic and not to supplemental benefits.

The conferees reduced mandatory benefits, but retained, at the Senate's request, alcoholism and drug abuse treatment. Supplemental services would be provided at an HMO's discretion. The mandatory dual-choice provision was modified to give employers with more than 25 employees a bit more flexibility: they would have to include an HMO in their health benefits plan only if employees lived within the HMO's service area. Employers retained the right not to offer an HMO option until approached by a federally qualified plan. Finally, the importance of collective bargaining agents was reaffirmed: they would have first right of refusal on an HMO option for their membership.

The Senate adopted the conference bill by voice-vote on September 16, and the House cleared the bill by a vote of 298-29 on September 23.

H.R.9019 went to President Gerald R. Ford's desk in early October, very close to Congress's adjournment for the fall elections. In fact, the bill was on the President's desk when adjournment came, raising the spectre of a possible pocket veto. As had happened so many times in the past, friends of HMO serendipitously appeared on the scene at a critical moment.

The Office of Management and Budget (OMB) had long displayed its hostility to HMOs by using the budgetary process to inhibit HMO growth and development. Now, these same enemies might have the last word. Fortunately, Spencer Johnson had moved over to the Domestic Council to head up the health policy division. And, even more fortuitously, John G. Veneman, who as HEW Under Secretary had launched the original HMO policy initiative six years earlier, was now the senior staff aide to the Domestic Council, as Vice-President Nelson Rockefeller's counselor.

Johnson and Veneman went to work for the HMO amendments. OMB presented numerous objections to the bill, primarily focusing on the broadening of the federal grants commitment beyond the original five-year demonstration period. These objections were brushed aside by

Johnson and Veneman. Ford signed the bill into law on October 8, 1976, as P.L.94-460.

The Carter Administration Rediscovers HMO

Paradoxes have a way of catching up with policy initiatives. On January 20, 1977, the Democrats returned to power in the executive branch, after eight years of Republican control. The event was not without its risks for the emerging HMO industry. Not that a health system reform of HMO's magnitude would be uncomfortable under Democratic stewardship. But each change in the national political arena meant a period of transition, when new friends would have to be found and made as old ones departed. For the HMO industry, the transition period was particularly difficult because of the almost constant turmoil of Public Health Service program management and White House-OMB-HEW/Office of the Secretary neglect, experienced since the advent of P.L.93-222.

How would the Carter Administration react to HMOs? Would the new Administration perceive HMO as a social reform that, all along, would have been better guided by the Democratic party? Or would it discard HMO as a Republican scheme to deflect interest away from national health insurance?

The answers to these questions would await the shaping of health initiatives by the new team. Meanwhile, a period of watchful waiting set in as the industry and the HMO health bureaucracy cast a somewhat uneasy eye toward the Georgians and their colleagues.

* * *

Soon after Jimmy Carter gained the Democratic nomination for President in July 1976, HMO lobbyists went to work to secure a position of visibility on the Democratic candidate's health policy agenda. Led by Group Health Association of America advocates, old friends of the HMO movement were approached — Max Fine, executive director of the Committee for National Health Insurance; former Rep. Roy, the architect of the original House HMO bill and an early Carter supporter; and Bert Seidman, head of the AFL-CIO Social Security Department.

These efforts proved successful. The Democratic candidate referred to HMOs in a speech before the National Medical Association and in a major address before the American Public Health Association in late October. After the election, a thoughtful position paper on HMOs was prepared for the Carter transition team by Joseph Onek, a Washington-based lawyer, who was executive director of the Center for Law and Social Policy, and Brian Biles, who wrote the original House HMO bill as a legislative aide to former Rep. Roy. Onek and Biles hoped to bring HMOs to the attention of the President-elect and HEW Secretary-designate, Joseph A. Califano Jr.

As had happened so many times previously, HMO got lost in a swamp of confusing and competing health policy priorities. In 1970, the ill-fated Health Options process had nearly buried the embryonic HMO initiative under a mountain of health policy proposals, all competing for position on President Richard M. Nixon's health policy agenda. In 1973, HMO fell victim to the benign neglect of Republican indifference in the White House and HEW Office of the Secretary, leaving the federal effort to an unworkable PHS administrative process. Now, in the late fall of 1976, HMO was ensnared in yet another trap: the chaotic Carter transition team process.

The problem was not the organization of the transition *per se,* but rather that the eight years just past had been years of frustration for many liberal health causes, which suffered at the hands of successive conservative Republican regimes. Particularly hard hit by the cutbacks of the early '70s had been the various categorical support programs for the poor that had blossomed in the late '60s and during the first Nixon term. Following the 1972 election, these programs suffered the full onslaught of Nixon's determination to reduce "extravagant" federal support of social and health programs.

The poor were not the only ones eager to plead their case. The myriad health professional organizations and categorical disease lobbies had also been frustrated by Republican attempts to bring a measure of budgetary coherence in such areas as health manpower and biomedical research. Now, these groups, too, wanted an opportunity to plead their special merits before the President-elect.

The transition teams were unwieldy potpourris of interest group representatives and individual job seekers, not the most favorable environments for in-depth study of complex proposals for health system reform. Such an environment of passion and confusion was a poor forum in which to put forward HMO as a comprehensive health system reform. Thus, HMO was never seriously considered by top leadership during the frenetic days preceding the inauguration.

The health priorities presented to Carter lacked coherent structure and organization. They were poorly packaged, which somewhat annoyed this most orderly of Presidents-elect. HMO was only a minor element in an array of choices, and the Onek-Biles HMO position paper never received a hearing. It was swallowed up in the competition for position on the President's early health policy agenda.

The new team of health policy makers assembled by Califano had no particular predisposition toward HMOs. There were, however, a few sympathetic members of the new team: Under Secretary Hale Champion had served as a member of the board of trustees of the Harvard Community Health Plan. Biles arrived from the transition team as a deputy of Karen Davis, the deputy assistant secretary for health planning; and Grant Spaeth, the new deputy assistant secretary for health legislation, was an attorney from California who had served as counsel to an HMO in the Palo Alto area.

The new Administration, however, began its search for health policies in much the same way as a different new Administration had eight years earlier. It began with a piece of the problem. Health care cost inflation was again perceived to be the immediate source of crisis. So in March 1977, the new Administration launched a major initiative to bring runaway hospital costs under control by seeking to impose a mandatory 9 percent ceiling on the annual inflation rate to be allowed hospitals. This would mean that, almost immediately, the rate would have to be reduced from a current annual level of 14 percent.

During the spring of 1977, HMO development chief Frank Seubold sent a memo to William Fullerton, deputy director of the newly established Health Care Financing Administration.[10] The memo pointed out that, in the long run, HMOs, by reducing inpatient utilization rates just 5 percent would save more money than the 9 percent cap on the hospital inflation rate. Therefore, HMOs should not be forgotten as HEW moved forward with its cost containment initiative. The memo had no perceptible impact on the structure of the cost containment initiative — although, as it turned out, HMOs were on the minds of a number of people advising the Secretary, particularly Spaeth. A re-connection between HMOs and cost containment was imminent.

An opportunity to move HMOs to the top of the policy agenda came in May, when Spaeth invited GHAA lobbyists in for a general discussion of HMOs. Significantly, Spaeth, as HEW's chief health legislation official, was then playing a pivotal role in the development of the hospital cost containment initiative, an effort requiring the drafting and submis-

10. HCFA brought the Medicare and Medicaid programs together for the first time, under one management structure — a long overdue reform.

sion of a hospital cost containment bill to the Congress. At their meeting, Spaeth pointed out that HMOs had been placed on the agenda of an upcoming briefing of Califano on recent departmental health initiatives. But, he noted, no specific recommendations had been prepared. Spaeth then asked GHAA's chief lobbyist Jim Doherty the critical question: "Do you have anything to get me on HMOs, particularly on hospital utilization and savings?

By coincidence, the Civil Service Commission had requested, a month or two earlier, that contractors issue statements on their plans and prospects of producing cost savings for the Federal Employees Health Benefits Program. It was a routine request, and the Kaiser Plans of California submitted the information, accompanied by a tabular presentation comparing national hospital utilization rates and costs under the fee-for-service system to the costs of such services as provided by the five Kaiser Plan hospitals. Doherty got this memo to Spaeth, in time for the Secretary's briefing.

Spaeth immediately saw the compelling significance of the Kaiser Plans' impact on hospital costs: 349 bed days/1,000 population (Kaiser) compared with 1,149 bed days/1,000 population (national average). There they were in the middle of a major cost containment initiative, and here was evidence of dramatic hospital cost reductions. When Califano asked for information about HMOs, Spaeth handed the Secretary the Kaiser-CSC memo. Upon seeing the hospital utilization rate table, Califano called for an immediate action memorandum on how HEW could vigorously move forward with an HMO initiative. This was a significant milestone in the checkered life of HMO as a federal health policy initiative. The Secretary's decision at that May briefing to move forward vigorously on HMOs was comparable in importance to the decision seven years earlier, in February 1970, to push HMOs as a cornerstone of Nixon Administration health policy. In a sense, HMOs had come full circle and were, once again, a national priority.

Events moved rapidly after this pivotal meeting with the Secretary. In early June, a briefing memorandum was prepared by Henry Aaron, the Assistant Secretary for Planning and Evaluation, and his staff.[11] That memo presented 12 recommendations for administrative actions to revitalize the floundering HMO program, which had never really recovered from the neglect suffered during the Nixon-Ford Administrations.

---

11. Health Maintenance Organizations, memorandum from the Assistant Secretary for Planning and Evaluation to the Secretary, HEW, June 3, 1977.

The recommended actions were:

- Public encouragement
- Speeding up of the qualification process
- Active promotion and technical assistance
- Issuing needed regulations
- Dual choice for Medicare
- Dual choice for Medicaid
- Revitalization of continuing compliance
- Reorganizing HEW operations affecting both development and qualification; legislative action required
- Extension of legislation
- Medicare and Medicaid HMO reimbursement
- Federal matching for Medicare HMOs
- Modification of qualification requirements

This list of proposed reforms was comprehensive. It addressed virtually every problem in HMO policy implementation that had been plaguing the HEW-based initiative since the program's earliest experiences under P.L.93-222. Also, it recognized, significantly, that the HMO statute, only recently amended in 1976, would again need to be amended, especially in view of the fact that the 1976 amendments had only extended the program an additional two years. Thus, HMO advocates would have further opportunities to refine the enabling authority into a workable instrument.

The decision to move vigorously on a renewed HMO initiative made sense for reasons other than the cost containment issue. Just over the horizon, there loomed an ominous report from the Senate oversight Committee on Governmental Affairs, highly critical of California's experience with enrolling the poor in HMO prototypes under Medicaid. Even though HEW had played no direct role in the ill-fated California prepaid health scandals, guilt by association was a very real possibility.[12] Therefore, HEW had to put some distance between itself and the previous Republican Administration's mishandling of the HMO program. In short, economic and political realities converged in June 1977, pointing to a re-establishment of HEW's leadership in the HMO arena, under the new Democratic Administration.

---

12. U.S. Congress. Senate. Committee on Government Affairs, Permanent Subcommittee on Investigations. *Prepaid Health Plans and Health Maintenance Organizations: A Report.* Senate Report No. 95-000. Washington, DC: U.S. Government Printing Office, 1978.

The opportunity to launch the new initiative came on June 20, 1977, when Champion delivered the keynote address to GHAA's annual Group Health Institute, held that year in Los Angeles. The Under Secretary took steps to place the blame for HEW's poor performance to date on prior Republican Administrations. He committed HEW to a seven-point program, designed to reverse the situation.[13] These were the commitments:

1. To encourage greater private investment in HMOs and to extend federal enabling legislation beyond 1978
2. To target future HMO development, supported by federal resources, among areas and with groups that have potential to form HMOs, and then to provide them with technical assistance
3. To reorganize the HEW HMO program and to ensure greater coordination between the grant and qualification program components
4. To reduce rapidly the backlog of applications for qualification
5. To speed up the promulgation of regulations
6. To enforce standards more vigorously among federally qualified HMOs to protect their subscribers
7. To increase Medicare and Medicaid enrollment in HMOs

The Under Secretary concluded his remarks in language meant to stir memories of past Democratic efforts to solve critical social problems:

> . . . let us together try to revive the confidence and enthusiasm of earlier years, to overcome the distrust and pessimism of the recent past — some of which seems to be carrying over to the present in Washington.
>
> . . . Attitudes will have to change and so will aspirations. But if we can rebuild mutual confidence in social progress . . . then we'll begin to actually make some again.[14]

The Under Secretary's final words were prophetic in light of events that followed: "I've given you a lot to hold us to."

* * *

---

13. Honorable Hale Champion, Under Secretary U.S. Department of Health, Education, and Welfare, "Keynote Address," in Proceedings, 27th Annual Group Health Institute, Los Angeles, CA, June 19-22, 1977, Washington, DC: Group Health Association of America, 1977, pp. 272-279.
14. *Ibid.*

Champion took charge of the new HMO initiative and placed day-to-day responsibility for implementing his seven-point program of action with Deputy Assistant Secretary for Health Joyce Lashof, M.D. Chief targets were a quick reduction of the backlog of applications in the qualification office, the search for a new director for the HMO program, and the commissioning of an outside review of HMO program structure and management.

During the summer of 1977, Milton I. Roemer, M.D., a professor of public health at UCLA and highly regarded in social medicine circles, intensively examined HMO program operations.[15] He concluded that a fundamental reorganization was required — one that would pull the development and qualification arms of the program together under a single administrative structure. Roemer also recommended that the newly reorganized entity be housed temporarily in the Office of the Assistant Secretary for Health, later to be relocated in the Health Resources Administration.

While internal HEW plans for reorganizing the HMO effort took shape, the Secretary and Under Secretary launched a highly visible series of activities, designed to communicate their seriousness of purpose to the skeptical health, business, and labor communities. The strategy was not without risk, for it irrevocably linked HEW prestige to the yet unresolved management issues that had plagued the HMO initiative from its inception.

The backlog of pending qualification applications was noticeably reduced by late fall. On October 27, Califano officially welcomed the largest HMO in the nation, the Kaiser Foundation Health Plan, into the ranks of qualified HMOs. Califano's speech, sponsored by the LBJ Foundation on the occasion of Kaiser's 40th anniversary, was designed to provide strong symbolic evidence that HMOs, products of the great social reforms of the 1930s, were now being embraced by those in direct line of descent from the New Deal and Great Society eras. Finally, in December, it was announced that Secretary Califano would sponsor a conference of business and industry leaders interested in HMO development, on March 10, 1978. The format was quickly broadened to include the organized labor movement, when old friends of the HMO movement from labor's ranks indicated, in no uncertain terms, that they would feel slighted if not included in the meeting.

---

15. Milton I. Roemer, M.D., Report on the Management of HMO Program, HEW, Aug. 1977.

These well-publicized activities, noteworthy for their clear signal that the Carter Administration was indeed serious about revitalizing the federal HMO initiative, overshadowed a less visible series of actions involving HEW's internal reorganization of the federal HMO program offices. Behind the scenes, there was less accomplishment than seemed to be indicated by the rhetoric of top HEW officials. By November, the search for a new HMO program director had bogged down. The Administration had initially sought to enlist the services of a physician with senior-level credentials in the HMO industry. This approach failed because it was impossible to entice such an individual from the established, high-paying security of a stable HMO into the lower paying uncertainty of an HMO bureaucracy in serious need of substantial reform.

At a November 15 status report briefing for the Under Secretary, it was clear that the reorganization process was in need of refocusing and firm leadership. Champion, for his part, had been apprised by HMO lobbyists that Schweiker would be seeking additional legislative amendments in early 1978. Moreover, both he and Califano had promised to produce visible and tangible results in short order. Clearly, extraordinary actions were called for. These followed swiftly on the heels of the November 15 meeting.

Champion placed HEW's floundering HMO initiative under the direct supervision of Leo Corbett, his executive assistant, and Bruce Wolff, a special assistant to the Secretary. Corbett convened a special HMO task force, issued assignments to both HMO staff in the bureaucracy and special members assigned from other agencies. The two warring program offices, HMO Development and HMO Qualification, were officially united in the Office of the Assistant Secretary for Health on January 15, 1978. The search for a new director of the combined program ended in February with the selection of Howard R. Veit, assistant commissioner of the Massachusetts Department of Public Health. Corbett and Wolff directly managed the new Office of HMOs from the Office of the Secretary until Veit assumed control in March.

The Legislative Prod: 1978 HMO Amendments

The launching of the new HMO initiative on March 1, 1978, eight months after Champion committed HEW to that course of action, was markedly accelerated by and coincided with a new round of legislative activity. Certainly, there was need for a program extension, if further appropriations were to be forthcoming. The development of a substantive set of proposals, moreover, served to move the process of HMO bureaucratic regeneration along. In the byzantine world of HEW health politics, one of the best ways to produce consensus is to force agencies and offices to draw together around the legislative process and to produce congressional testimony for the Secretary. Hospital cost containment legislation had provided the needed stimulus to prod HEW to rediscover obvious cost containment implications of HMOs. In the fall, it was the early prospect of congressional action on HMOs that, once again, prodded HEW's sluggish bureaucracy to further efforts at rehabilitating the HMO initiative.

HMO lobbyists, as well as top HEW officials, knew that as soon as a bill was filed and hearings scheduled, the Office of Management and Budget would approach HEW for its position. The need to respond to OMB, in turn, would create the necessary stimulus to move the HMO initiative forward.

The strategy was launched with the knowledge of senior HEW officials, and, in early December, Schweiker announced at the winter meeting of the GHAA Group Health Institute that he would soon be filing a bill to accomplish 10 objectives:[16]

1. Extension of the authorization
2. Broadened flexibility and secretarial discretion in financing and qualifying HMOs
3. Periodic restatement of goals and purposes of the HMO program by the executive branch
4. Increased ceilings on grants and loans
5. Expansion grants for further development of qualified HMOs and grants and/or loans to meet additional capital requirements
6. Medicare and Medicaid amendments to gain meaningful participation of the elderly and poor
7. Establishment of a federal mechanism to protect individuals, if nonqualified HMOs fail
8. Exemption of HMOs from the certificate-of-need requirements under P.L.93-641, the National Health Planning and Resources Development Act
9. Stronger protection against fraud, abuse, and self-dealing
10. Authorization of HEW to unify its administration of the HMO program

---

16. Remarks of Sen. Richard S. Schweiker, Group Health Institute, Washington, DC: Dec. 12, 1977.

Schweiker introduced his promised amendments on February 10, 1978, as S.2534, the Health Maintenance Organization Amendments of 1978. The Administration submitted its own bill shortly thereafter, and Rogers introduced a House version, H.R.13266, on June 22.

Hearings on these bills were held in the House and Senate during the spring and summer of 1978. The Senate reported S.2534 on June 22, and the House reported a clean, marked up bill, H.R.13655, on July 31. S.2534 passed the Senate on July 21, and H.R. 13655 passed the House on September 25. The House and Senate agreed to the conference report on October 13 and 14, respectively. Carter signed P.L.95-559, the Health Maintenance Organization Amendments of 1978, on November 1.

In addition to extending HMO program authorizations for three years, the amendments increased the maximum dollar limit for initial development project grants, contracts, and loan guarantees from $1 million to $2 million. A new category of expansion grants was also established, as was a new management intern program authority. Another set of provisions dealt with the regulatory aspects of the HMO program by tightening financial disclosure and enrollment practice requirements.

The National HMO Development Strategy: Managing an Emerging Industry

The passage of the 1978 HMO amendments, combined with the renewed commitment of the Carter Administration to HMO development, set the stage for a period of rapid growth and expansion of HMOs. The President's fiscal year 1980 budget, one of the most austere ever to be proposed by a Democratic President, nevertheless requested $74 million for the HMO program, more than twice the requested appropriation for fiscal year 1979 of $31 million. Congress subsequently authorized a fiscal year 1980 appropriation of $48 million. The renewed commitment also meant that the HMO program would aggressively promote the development of new HMOs by focusing on locations with good growth potential and then coordinating resource investments in those areas.

During the early part of 1979, HEW launched its national HMO development strategy, based on the concept of "community targeting." HEW noted that the targeting approach represented a departure from the more restrained approach of past Administrations, which waited for applicants to come forward from communities without actively stimulating developmental efforts in specific locations.[17] The objective of the new

17. See: National HMO Development Strategy, through 1988, HEW, Office of Health Maintenance Organizations, 1979.

strategy was to maximize the community cost savings potential of HMOs by stimulating their development in those areas of the country experiencing the highest levels of health care cost inflation. Twenty locations with the highest health care costs in 1978 were selected as the first priority, while other locations with high HMO growth potential and somewhat lower costs were also selected. In all, 61 target areas were chosen, each being a standard metropolitan statistical area (SMSA).

The new strategy committed the federal government to a 10-year program of sustained support for HMOs, at the end of which there would be:

- 442 HMOs, an increase of 239 over the 1978 total of 203
- 19.1 million enrollees, an increase of 11.7 million over the 1978 total of 7.4 million
- Approximately $20.3 billion in community cost savings resulting from HMOs' operations during this 10-year period

These growth projections, while far more sober than those offered in 1971, when 1,700 HMOs were forecast by 1977, had the benefit of hindsight not available in those early years. The nearly 10 years of experience with active federal commitment clearly argued for conservative forecasts, which, nonetheless, offered the nation substantial benefits, particularly in cost savings.

The new development strategy also anticipated a significant increase in privately funded HMOs, about nine per year, or 90 between 1978 and 1988. This estimate would yield about half as many privately funded HMOs as those funded through federal investments. The health insurance industry, in particular, appeared ready to make a significant commitment to HMO development, while industry and labor also expressed renewed interest.

The challenge of the 1980s appeared to be one of managing growth, perhaps an even more complex undertaking than earlier challenges involving a basic fight for survival. In this context, the federal government would have to face new questions about its role in the rapidly maturing HMO industry:[18]

---

18. As this book went to press, concern was mounting in high-level governmental and HMO industry circles that HEW's managerial control of the HMO program had not yet caught up with Carter Administration rhetoric and substantial budgetary commitments. As the tempo of developmental activities increased dramatically in 1978 and 1979, thoughtful analysts began to look uneasily at both HEW's HMO administrative infrastructure and at the capabilities of new applicants for federal grant assistance. Of particular concern was the steady increase in the number of insolvencies among newer

- Should federal investments be phased out, if and when private investments increased substantially?
- Was there any real possibility at all that private industry would make a serious financial commitment to establishing prepaid health plans?
- As the federal government moved forward with its own plans to market HMOs aggressively in target areas, how would private HMO developers respond, such as insurance companies? Would they take the competitive bait? Or, would they shy away from the challenge?
- As the industry rapidly expanded, could it manage its own growth, in terms of financial stability and quality of service, or would the federal government be required to establish an elaborate HMO regulatory system to police the entire program?
- Would sophisticated managerial talent take charge of HMO development in order to ensure that rapid growth was not accompanied by a large number of HMO failures?[19]

The answers to these questions were far from certain in mid-1979. The only certainty appeared to be the permanence of HMOs as viable alternatives to fee-for-service health care.

HMOs, suggesting the marginal nature of many of the plans funded through federal grants and loans over the past three years. It appeared certain that a renewed period of reflection and evaluation about the future federal role was in the offing.

19. The scarcity of technically qualified management personnel throughout the industry was recognized by the Congress through the passage, with the 1978 HMO amendments, of authorization for a national HMO management training program. The federal Office of HMOs also recognized that there was a general lack of HMO management skills among its permanently employed (federal) work force. Therefore, during the fall of 1979, the Office of HMOs commissioned private contracts to develop training curriculums and to conduct seminars and training programs for its large staff, in a major effort to upgrade their professional skills levels.

CHAPTER 8

HMOs and the Future of Health System Reform

With the reorganization of the HMO program in the Public Health Service, the 1978 legislative amendments, and the launching of a new national HMO development strategy, the most recent chapter in the saga of HMO has come to a close. It is a logical place to close this book, as well. This final chapter, therefore, reviews the progress of the past eight years, describes present challenges, and looks to the future.[1]

The Changing HMO Marketplace

That HMOs have made progress in gaining a respectable position in the mainstream of American health care cannot be denied. In 1929, when the Ross-Loos Clinic opened its doors in Los Angeles, at about the time Michael Shadid, M.D., established the Elk City (Oklahoma) Cooperative, these were the only two prepaid health plans in the nation. In 1970, there were 39 prepaid plans with 3.6 million people enrolled. Then came the active commitment of the federal government.

1. Data in this chapter are drawn from studies conducted by HEW's Office of HMO as part of its efforts to develop the national HMO development strategy. See: National HMO Development Strategy, through 1988, HEW/Office of HMO, 1979. Also see: "Estimates of HMO Growth and Related Cost Savings, 1978-90," ICF, Inc. Feb. 1979.

Causal inference in the social sciences still remains a mixture of science and art. In a field as dynamic as health policy development, there is a special need to tread cautiously and to avoid bold claims. Having duly noted the hazards of prediction, it is still reasonable to highlight startling associations: from 1970 through mid-1979, the number of HMOs grew from 39 to 217 and HMO enrollment doubled from 3.6 million to 7.9 million persons. Certainly, it is not unreasonable, at first glance, to associate the federal government's active intervention with these dramatic increases.

The question is: In what ways has the federal government influenced progress in the HMO marketplace? There are three possible answers to this question:

- Federal intervention has facilitated the growth and development of HMOs.
- Federal intervention has inhibited the growth and development of HMOs.
- Federal intervention has accomplished both: it has simultaneously facilitated and inhibited HMO growth and development.

The third possibility offers the most reasonable explanation. On the one hand, federal dollars and publicity have stimulated HMO development. On the other hand, congressional insistence on shaping the emerging universe of HMOs to a set of rigid specifications, coupled with persistent executive branch difficulties in administering so complex a program, has inhibited the HMO industry's maturation. This conclusion has been amply documented in preceeding pages of this book.

It should be emphasized, however, that simple moral judgments about the federal role do a disservice to matters not so easily evaluated. For example, a thoughtful observer of health care systems might well conclude that the elaborate federal requirements for qualification, established in Section 1310 of the HMO Act, are entirely justifiable as minimal standards to ensure quality and consumer protection. Other observers, however, might conclude that the federal government should not intrude so heavily into the structuring of HMOs, allowing market forces to shape the minimum scope of benefits, organizational forms, and enrollment policies. Everyone seems to agree that health care markets do not spontaneously produce innovations unless stimulated by philanthropic or public investments. Analysts divide sharply, however, on how the positive incentive of investments ought to be balanced with the negative reinforcement of regulations.

A significant amount of HMO developmental activity has been stimulated by federal investments in three regions of the country: rapid expansions of HMOs have occurred throughout California, in the upper Midwest, and along the East Coast. Thus, between 1970 and 1978, 25 new HMOs became operational in California, 41 came on line in the five states comprising HEW's Region V, and 19 became operational in New England and the Middle Atlantic states. These three areas — California, the Upper Midwest, and the East Coast — account for 50 percent of the new HMOs since 1970. In short, HMOs have taken hold in the largest standard metropolitan statistical areas: 55 SMSAs, in all, encompassing 35 states, the District of Columbia, and Guam.

One way to determine the extent to which federal restrictiveness might have dampened HMO development is to look at the association between the rate of development of new HMOs and visible shifts in federal policy. Such an analysis must recognize the lag time between the beginning of an HMO development project and its movement into operation, an elapsed time averaging about three years. Thus, policy shifts affecting HMO development can be seen taking effect in the market about three years hence.

Two policy shifts occurred between 1970 and 1978 that could be interpreted as depressing to HMO development. First, there was the Nixon Administration's retreat from earlier commitments to HMOs, beginning in mid-1972, along with congressional insistence that pre-Act new starts be halted. Second, there were the combined effects, following enactment of P.L.93-222 of (a) Congress's restrictive definitions of HMOs, along with (b) the Ford Administration's delays in promulgation of mandatory dual-choice regulations, and (c) their determination to restrict the HMO development budget severely, limiting grant support of new starts (feasibility studies) in fiscal year 1977 to only five projects.

The data show that these policy shifts did, in fact, contribute to an overall slowdown in HMO growth. Between 1970 and 1974, the number of operating HMOs increased from 39 to 163 — an increase of 124 new HMOs. Between 1974 and 1978, the number of HMOs grew to 203 — only 40 new HMOs. Forty-six of the new plans emerging between 1970 to 1974 came from California, whereas over the next four years, California lost 21 plans. Even with the retrenchment in California factored out, it is clear that growth in the 1974-78 period was much slower than in the previous four-year period.

What If?

The foregoing review presented a close-up of HMO development. Although it accurately portrayed the evolving HMO marketplace and suggested possible associations with federal policy, a more profound question might be asked: Could the dramatic forecasts of HMO development, offered in 1971 by the enthusiastic band of HMO advocates in HEW, have been sustained if the federal government had fully committed itself to the HMO concept? Would the 1,700 HMOs promised in 1971 have become a reality in 1977?

The answer to such a speculative question requires one to posit the following further questions:

- What if the White House had sustained its enthusiasm for HMOs?
- What if the reimbursement mechanism that was enacted under Section 1876 of the Social Security Act in 1972 had been favorable to prepaying HMOs in their accustomed manner?
- What if national health insurance had been enacted?
- What if the federal government had established strict price controls over particular sectors of the health system, for example, physicians, hospitals?
- What if unlimited federal funds had been available, in concert with one or more of the alternatives just proposed?

These questions are reminiscent of the kind of "thinking about the unthinkable" that brought futurologist Herman Kahn such notoriety in the early 1960s when he speculated on *what if* nuclear warfare became a reality. Such speculations invariably upset someone or other, primarily because the requirements of *what if* forecasting necessitate changing the balance of history and politics. Thus, to speculate on *what ifs* affecting the past nine years of HMO experience requires us to assume some startling revisions in the recent history of health care politics:

- Republican Administrations would have remained steadfast in their commitment to what had always been a liberal social reform.
- The Senate Finance Committee and the Social Security Administration would have accepted the logic of fixed-price prepayment and changed their behavior accordingly.
- Sen. Edward M. Kennedy (D-MA) and his health aide, Philip Caper, M.D., would have accepted prevailing HMO industry guidelines of HMO benefit packages, enrollment procedures, and premium structures, rather than imposing upon them their normative vision of the future alternative health care delivery system.
- National health insurance would have become available to provide a ready source of payment for HMOs. The competitive advantage of the monopolistic health insurance industry and fee-for-service medicine could have been effectively neutralized.

- Federal anti-inflationary price controls would have created substantial incentives among health care providers to seek more cost efficient ways of delivering health care.
- The congressional appropriations committees and the Office of Management and Budget would have provided the HMO program all of the venture capital it required to take advantage of dramatically changing market conditions.

Had these environmental conditions prevailed over the previous decade, the development of HMOs would certainly have been accelerated. Even during the earlier period of less than enthusiastic support, there was significant private sector interest in HMO development. Of the 203 plans that had become operational by 1978, 121 of them were started without benefit of federal grants or loans. It is reasonable to conclude, therefore, that greater federal interest during the 1970s would have stimulated an even more enthusiastic response from the private sector.

The Politics of HMO

The relevance of such *what if* speculation is to highlight the inevitable gap between performance and possibility. Each of our speculative *what ifs* assumed away the most important issue of all: the negative politics that HMO reform proposals have stimulated. Our speculation, of course, finessed the obvious point that health maintenance proposed not just the ends of health care reform, a nationwide network of cost efficient HMOs, but also the means of reform, a series of concrete actions that the federal government would take to achieve the objective of high HMO growth by the end of the 1970s.

The spectre of a truly competitive network of HMOs directly threatened the economic independence of the nation's physicians, galvanizing the AMA to strong opposition. The possible precedent of using large outlays of public funds to subsidize these reforms motivated fiscal conservatives in the Congress to oppose a substantial federal development program. The threat of major revisions to the "usual, customary, and reasonable" cost and fee reimbursement mechanisms that undergird the Medicare bureaucracy and its ever watchful patron, the Senate Finance Committee, neutralized the potential leverage favorable to HMOs that the largest federal health program could have had. Even stalwart HMO advocates began to waver in their support, as the federal program started to take shape far to the left of what they believed that plans already in operation, or those not yet begun, could tolerate.

HMOs, in short, were significant enough reforms in prevailing health care practice to trouble nearly everyone. However, like all well-conceived social reforms, HMOs offered enough positive benefits to enough opponents to effectively fragment the opposition. Thus, the federal commitment prevailed through a classic compromise of American democratic politics: the left (Kennedy) and right (AMA) neutralized each other, enabling the center (the HMO advocacy) to achieve sufficient consensus to pass a piece of legislation minimally unsatisfactory to everyone. Of course, P.L.93-222 was unworkable from the first precisely because it compromised the uncompromisable and reconciled the irreconcilable. The full measure of this burden immediately fell upon the Public Health Service bureaucracy. The 1976 HMO amendments undid much of the initial mischief caused by the 1973 compromise, and the 1978 amendments substantially completed the task.

No politics comparable to the HMO advocacy, responsible for legislative progress, is available to sustain a politics of implementation. HMOs do not have a natural grass-roots constituency, in the classic manner of American interest group politics, to champion their causes in communities and in the federal health bureaucracies. The 217 extant plans are not yet a political force, and significant conflicts exist among them, most notably the natural antipathy of prepaid group practice plans for IPAs and vice versa.

The HMO advocacy is strongest in the Congress, at the point where the ardor of a few can be truly amplified, that is, in the authorizing health committees. HMOs do well in these key committees because of their persuasive logic, not because of the power behind their advocacy. When the focus shifts to other matters, for example, appropriations and oversight of HMO operations, the enemies of HMO are able to marshal formidable weaponry. Then, the logic of HMO as an abstract health care reform must meet the challenge of operational performance. Like most innovations, the record shows pluses and minuses; on the whole, the pluses win out. But in the hostile forums of certain congressional subcommittees, the defense is often silent.

There are a number of reasons why HMOs generally have a rough time with congressional committees beyond the authorizing health subcommittees. First, HMOs concretely threaten powerful entrenched interests in the health care establishment while offering primarily abstract benefits to consumers of health care, for example, health care cost savings to consumers that pay for few health care services out of pocket; reduced days of hospitalization, which neither patients nor physicians find particularly significant but which assuredly agitates hospital administrators; and, most intangible of all, "wellness." Such intangibles are rarely the mainstays of practical politics. Physicians threatened by HMO competition know their interests are at stake. Consumers paying for health care out of a monthly premium deduction are only marginally affected. In fact, their actual premium charges will probably be the same, or even somewhat higher than comparable premiums for Blue Cross or indemnity plans. The fact that HMO benefits are substantially broader is another bothersome abstraction.

Second, the implementation of the HMO development program in the Public Health Service does not, *ipso facto,* ensure a vocal constituency of supportive grantees in the nation's communities. Unlike neighborhood health center and community mental health center grant programs, the HMO development grant process is arduous and complex. Many who begin at the feasibility study level (at least 50 percent) fail to make it to the planning level. And, having successfully invested three years in planning and development, the newly operating plan must struggle to break even within five years in order to begin repaying federal loans.

Tension and conflict between the federal bureaucracy, venture capitalizing the process, and local developers are built into the system. Inevitably, unhappy grantees who have been terminated after a particular development phase, or who are desperately awaiting a transfusion of needed cash, will complain to their congressmen about their difficulties with the bureaucracy. The emergence of a comprehensive qualification and compliance process, in response to congressional calls for more vigorous monitoring of operating HMOs, can only amplify these tensions and conflicts.

Moreover, the nature of the federal role, both as investor and as regulator, creates ambivalence among potential HMO constituents. Once a plan is in full operation and has received its federal qualification certificate, it has little interest in the federal program. In fact, as one candid plan director has put it:

> Strictly from the viewpoint of self-interest, after we've used federal dollars to become established, we have little interest in being regulated. We certainly don't relish new federally sponsored projects threatening us with competition. There is little to compel us to form a supportive constituency for the federal program.

The large, established plans, such as Kaiser, speak for themselves in the political process. The Kaiser plans, in fact, have their own lobbying office in Washington, DC. The national HMO organizations, Group Health Association of America and the American Association of Foundations for Medical Care, do not yet represent unified constituencies. By May 1979, 91 of the 217 operating plans had become federally qualified, and it appeared inevitable that before long most of the plans would seek federal qualification. The political challenge was clear: to organize these well-established plans into a powerful grass-roots constituency that could champion the HMO cause not only during times of legislative amendment but also on a sustaining basis. This challenge would test the mettle of the two national leadership organizations over the decade of the 1980s.

Coming Full Circle

HMOs attract liberal health care reformers because they offer substance to the cause of health care reorganization. HMOs attract fiscal conservatives because they deliver health care at a lower cost than other systems of health care. For a time, in the early 1970s, the most ambitious liberals tried to load upon HMOs the extra burdens of a broad array of long-sought systemic reforms. Their impatience was understandable precisely because liberal health care reformers have been extraordinarily patient ever since the cause of national health insurance was first lost in 1935. Forty years of patience justifies, to some, the view that HMOs should be used as expedient instruments to achieve the aspirations of nearly half a century.

The economic situation in 1979 is much less clear than the situation in 1972. Now, it is not at all certain when national health insurance will be enacted. Most proponents agree it will not come before 1983. Robbed of the integrating framework of NHI, the liberal reformer has begun to take HMOs for precisely what they are, and not for what they might foreshadow. Under the right circumstances, HMOs can create climates of competition in health care markets long characterized by entrenched professional monopoly.[2] A curious "coming full circle," therefore, joins the advocates of the health maintenance strategy in 1970 to the HMO ad-

---

2. Recent experiences show that HMOs can stimulate intense competition in health care environments. For example, in Boston, Minneapolis-St. Paul, Detroit, and Boise, Idaho, multiple HMOs are locked in fierce competition both with traditional fee-for-service providers, the health insurance industry, and each other, in order to attract consumers to their plans. Although the data remain highly tentative, it appears, so far, that these competitive pressures are significantly affecting health care costs in these marketplaces, in a positive way. See: "Selected Use of Competition by HSAs," final report to HEW/Bureau of Health Planning and Resource Development, ICF, Inc., Dec. 1976.

vocates of 1979. In 1970, Republican reformers saw HMO as a necessary and major first-step reform that would be required to bring cost efficiency to health care systems. National health insurance, so important an agenda item for liberal Democrats, would have to wait until the inflation-wracked health sector of the economy could be brought under control. In 1979, events have brought the Republican strategy home to the incumbent Democratic Administration. HMOs and other cost containment measures have replaced NHI as the central elements of health system reform.

HMO: The Public Use of Private Interest

HMOs have survived a decade of trials that have proved them desirable and durable health system reforms. Without benefit of major allies in powerful, entrenched sectors of the health system and against substantial efforts to destroy the federal commitment, HMOs have emerged, in 1979, as the most available and expedient tool to achieve some measure of health system reform in the 1980s. National health insurance remains a distant promise. National health planning continues to flounder amid a confusion of objectives and the near impossibility of implementation. Hospital cost containment awaits an as yet to be achieved consensus among the Congress, Administration, and hospital interests.

HMOs remain viable instruments of reform, while other programs flounder. HMOs are unambiguous in purpose, amenable to concrete plans for implementation, and arouse less opposition than other reforms. Moreover, HMOs do not juxtapose the federal government in open conflict with health system components, but rather offer health systems the opportunity to shape their own futures. As pressures build for more objectionable change, the reasonableness of HMOs come home to broad elements of the health system. In short, HMOs are alternative models of health care organization that meet two basic requirements for reform in a pluralist democracy: they work, and private health interests find them increasingly acceptable.

If HMOs represent a concrete form of health system reform, then a public policy based on the objective of developing HMOs can be given scope with relative ease. Once the objective of HMO development is accepted by government, the specific steps that government must take also become clear. Thus, the ends of HMO development point to the means of orderly public policies. These policies all share one element that distinguishes them from other reforms: HMO implementation policies essentially are aimed toward stimulating innovation in privately organized health systems. HMOs are private organizations that offer opportunities for health system reform without excessive federal control. At this writing, even the qualification and compliance aspects of the federal HMO program have not yet become so burdensome as to overwhelm fledgling plans. In fact, the 1976 HMO amendments significantly reduced the comprehensiveness of requirements leading to qualification.[3] Coupled with effective technical assistance, federal regulation of HMOs can serve the highly constructive function of maintaining a high level of minimum standards for new plans to achieve and for older plans to maintain.

* * *

There was a time, in the early 1970s, when it seemed possible that HMOs could, by themselves, solve the problem of health care cost inflation. But more sober voices, principally from within the HMOs themselves, pleaded that HMOs were a part of a larger solution and not the solution itself. This matter emerged again in 1978, when failure to achieve significant progress in other areas of health system reform focused attention once again on HMOs.

Being the focus of national attention creates at least four possibilities. First, it means the availability of substantial development resources with which to plan the rapid growth of HMOs. Second, it means accepting burdens of public responsibility not levied on other health system sectors. HMOs must meet stipulations of federal law not required of solo practice physicians, fee-for-service groups, or hospitals. Third, attention means that other threatened sectors of the health system could be galvanized to attack HMOs. Reform usually provokes reaction. And fourth, national attention means that, in the absence of other appropriate health reforms, federal policymakers might well attempt to build an entire national health care reform strategy around HMOs.

---

3. This statement, of course, must be placed in proper perspective. P.L.93-222, as amended, does have complex rules that must be followed. They are, however, reasonably uncomplicated and unambiguous when compared to other federal health programs. Of course, critics of the federal effort continue to seek even less complexity of benefits, organizational forms, and premium structures. The 1976 amendments, however, brought the federal law substantially back to a position of flexibility and responsiveness to market reality.

These challenges present both opportunities and constraints. They represent the challenges of growth and prosperity, not of failure. Substantial resources for development make it necessary to plan growth wisely. HEW has set such a course with the launching of its national HMO development strategy in early 1979. Increased attention to quality assurance and financial viability have also become high priorities of the federal effort.

In the long run, HMOs will save significant amounts of money over comparable fee-for-service health care delivery systems. The matter of how quickly HMOs develop and expand, beyond their present numbers of 217 plans enrolling 7.9 million people, depends on forces outside the HMO industry and federal HMO program. The issue is one of incentive: how significant, over the coming years, third-party reimbursement mechanisms become in driving other health system components to seek the HMO alternative.

For example, if hospitals must reduce their costs, they may find the HMO attractive as a mechanism to extract significant economies from emergency rooms and outpatient departments. Solo practice physicians overburdened by malpractice insurance and the ever increasing costs of running their practices, may see the HMO as a viable means of reducing overhead.

In both cases, hospitals and physicians would be more rapidly propelled toward HMOs by mandatory federal price controls or the passage of a hospital cost containment bill. Such strong federal action was unthinkable in 1970; then came President Richard M. Nixon's Phase 2 price controls, which singled out hospitals and physicians for mandatory restraints. The period between 1971 and 1974, when Phases 1 and 2 were in effect, was the only period over the past two decades when health care price inflation was restrained. If federal policymakers secure congressional passage of mandatory hospital cost containment, a natural incentive for HMO formation will have been created among the nation's hardpressed hospital systems.

*   *   *

Charles L. Schultze, President Jimmy Carter's chief economic adviser, noted in the 1977 Godkin lectures at Harvard:

> Across a wide range of areas, social intervention often fails, not because it relies unnecessarily on regulation or other command-and-control devices, but because in other ways it ignores the roles

> of properly structured economic incentives for achieving social goals.[4]

Schultze's argument presents a compelling challenge to the federal health establishment to review carefully the types of regulations it promulgates in terms of desired outcomes in private economies. Schultze would recognize HMOs as constructive mechanisms of federal intervention. He would likewise criticize aspects of many of the federal intervention strategies that have preceded HMOs. Categorical grant programs, from Hill-Burton to Neighborhood Health Centers, helped fragment and maldistribute local health resources. Medicare and Medicaid paid for services without regard for the resulting negative impacts on local health system pricing structures. Comprehensive health planning and its lineal descendant, health planning and resources development, sought to rationalize and limit health resources deployment through an ineffectual patchwork of federal, state, and local health planning agencies.

Each of these programs has fallen short in one way or another. Federal resource production programs overproduced and maldistributed health resources. Medicare and Medicaid fueled inflation by supplying these resources with a greatly increased flow of dollars, and the health planning programs sought rationalization by seeking voluntary, noncoercive ways to control growth. HMOs, however, use public investments solely to provide venture capital to communities and local health systems seeking to reorganize themselves. There are no coercive elements to the HMO reform. Nor do HMOs appeal to more than the enlightened economic self-interest of health care components.

* * *

The next decade offers great promise for HMOs. By 1988, if present federal policies and likely private sector responses hold firm, there is a reasonable prospect of over 440 operating HMOs, offering health services to over 19 million people. The cumulative impact of this growth will yield over $20 billion in cost savings, dollars that would have otherwise been wastefully spent. The promise of these savings cannot be ignored. And the potential health benefits of a more rational health care delivery system, modeled on the HMO concept, are too precious to forfeit through a failure of vision or will.

---

4. Charles L. Schultze. *The Public Use of Private Interest.* Washington, DC: The Brookings Institution, 1977, p. 63.

Index